FIT OR FAT?

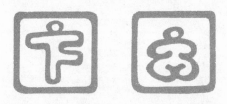

FIT OR FAT?®

Covert Bailey

With a Foreword by Joan Ullyot, M.D.

Houghton Mifflin Company / Boston

for Mina

For information about permission to reproduce selections from
this book, write to Permissions, Houghton Mifflin Company,
2 Park Street, Boston, Massachusetts 02108.

Library of Congress Cataloging in Publication Data

Bailey, Covert.
Fit or fat?
1. Reducing exercises. 2. Aerobic exercises.
3. Exercise — Physiological aspects. 4. Body
composition. I. Title.
RA781.6.B34   613.7′1   78-9757
ISBN 0-395-27161-4
ISBN 0-395-51083-X (pbk.)

Printed in the United States of America

Q 44 43 42 41 40 39 38 37 36

Fit or Fat® is a registered trademark of Covert Bailey.

Foreword

THERE IS an old saying to the effect that a person has perfect taste if it matches your own. In a similar vein, I believe that *Fit or Fat?* is the perfect book — it corroborates all my pet ideas about diets and exercise. These weighty topics occupy an enormous segment of the collective American consciousness. Theories abound and books proliferate, all promising the greatest girth control with the least amount of effort.

Covert Bailey takes a different approach. Not weight, but fat is the enemy. Not passive nutritional manipulations, but active changes in metabolism are the solution. Bailey's theories are based on experience as well as biochemical and nutritional analysis. The author, whose slim build and gargantuan appetite were the envy of his friends for years, was shocked one day to discover that fat had crept up on him unheralded. Realizing that the insidious onset of his problem coincided with a marked decrease in activity, he put two and two together (a simple matter for an M.I.T. graduate).

Boyish figure restored, Covert Bailey went on to spread the word around unfit America, in lectures and with his mobile "Bailey Clinic." *Fit or Fat?,* the resulting book, gives a lucid and entertaining explanation of the relationship between physical activity, fat metabolism, and weight. It includes sound nutritional advice based on these biochemical realities.

One's tendency, after reading this book, is to buy a dozen copies and distribute them to friends of both the fit and the fat variety. A little caution is recommended here. Many of the pudgy will be inspired to throw away their latest diets and calorie charts and go out for long walks or jogs, thus cluttering up the running paths. And Bailey's answers may not always please the already fit. My own charming, kind, and athletic uncle, an avid golfer all his life, read *Fit or Fat?* with tremendous enjoyment and murmurs of praise and approbation — until he learned that Bailey equated golf with canasta, in terms of exercise value. Whereupon he hurled the book across the room, with indignant curses. He was not sufficiently mollified to pick it up and finish it for several days.

Give the book to your friends anyway and strike a blow for improved fitness and health in America. This entertaining and enlightening book is the best way to dispel the myths of dieting and rescue millions of Americans from the pain of being "overfat," while liberating them from the tyranny of the bathroom scales.

JOAN ULLYOT, M.D.

San Francisco, 1978

Contents

	Foreword by Joan Ullyot, M.D.	v
1	Fat People Eat Less Than Skinny People	1
2	Diets Do Not Work	2
3	The Body Machine	4
4	Fat Floats!	6
5	Overweight versus Overfat	10
6	What Is Your Correct Weight?	14
7	What Is the Cure for All This Fat?	17
8	How Hard Should I Exercise?	23
9	If Two Aspirins Are Good, Four Must Be Better	29
10	How to Take an Exercise Pulse	32
11	Choosing an Aerobic Exercise	36
12	Heart Recovery after Exercise	46
13	Change in Muscle Shape	48
14	Should I Exercise When I Feel Ill?	50
15	Spot Reducing	53
16	Weight Lifting	57
17	Don't Confuse Work with Exercise	59
18	Insensible Exercise	61
19	Sing Praises to Protein	65
20	Do Muscles Burn Fat or Glucose?	71
21	Is There Anything Good about Fat Storage?	77

22 Fasting   81

23 People Are Eating Too Much Carbohydrate! Right?   83

24 How Much Fat Are Americans Eating?   87

25 The Big Picture   89

26 Muscle, Its Enzymes, and Mitochondria   94

27 Insulin Insensitivity   96

28 Contradictory Advice   98

29 Why Not Now?   100

    The Aerobics Logbook   103

1

Fat People Eat Less Than Skinny People

MOST FAT PEOPLE feel guilty! Society points its finger in shame at the overweight, making them feel that they are somehow morally weak, that they are gluttons with little strength of character. They chastise themselves at every meal, certain that they are overeating again. Nothing could be further from the truth. The will power of fat people never ceases to amaze me. They live a life of perpetual self-denial. If naturally skinny people denied themselves the way fat people do, they would fade away completely.

The truth is most fat people eat less than skinny people.

During the initial interview in our clinic, fat women quickly tell us that they know why they are fat. They are convinced that they eat too much. When we ask the typical fat lady if she eats more than other people, she answers that she eats more than anyone. But when we ask her about her husband's eating habits, she explodes in exasperation, "That darn man eats three or four helpings at every meal and is still as skinny as a beanpole!" About this time she recognizes her inconsistency. Her husband eats far more than she does. She may then insist that she snacks during the day, which is probably the truth. Most nutritionists (who ought to know better) believe that this is in fact the cause of her problem. But studies have confirmed that fat people are usually quite restrictive in their diets; that they eat less than their skinny spouses. The simple truth is that fat people have internal chemistry that has adapted to low-calorie intake. And when they *do* overindulge, as all of us do from time to time, they gain weight while their skinny friends stay slim.

2

Diets Do Not Work

IT'S ALMOST IMPOSSIBLE to read anything these days without finding another diet staring you in the face. At the supermarket checkout, there are the inevitable ladies' magazines, each with a brandnew diet, guaranteed to make you slim forever. The magazine racks are filled with new books with bright covers pushing new diets, and they too guarantee that you can become a Twiggy. There must be ten new, supposedly foolproof diets promoted every day. Usually the book makes claim — in bold type where you will be sure to see it — that you can eat all you want of the foods you like. After all, who wants to read about a new diet that expects you to give up good foods when that's what you are probably doing already?

Well, you can take heart, because the diets that tell you to give up the foods you like don't work. They don't work because none of the diets work. It should be obvious that when ten new diets are published every day, each one claiming to be perfect, that there is something fishy going on. The problem is that diets don't work in the first place. There is no diet now, and there never will be a diet that cures an overweight problem. The reason for this is that diets don't attack the fundamental problem of the fat person.

You see, most people think that losing weight is the basic problem. The fat person says, "I just can't lose weight." But when you ask the typical fat person if he has lost weight on any of the diets, he will tell you of the 30 pounds he lost on this diet, and the 20 pounds he lost on that. In fact, many of the patients that I have interviewed have lost 1000 pounds on various dietary programs over the years. Now, clearly, losing weight was not their problem at all. In fact, most fat people make a profession of losing weight.

They not only lose weight very easily but on practically every diet they try.

Sure, diets help people to lose weight; but losing weight is not the basic problem. The problem is — gaining weight! Fat people gain weight easily and quickly, so that they soon have more fat than they have just lost. Someone once said, "The American public has been dieting for twenty-five years — and has gained five pounds." Fat people who are constantly dieting should be asking themselves, "Why do I gain weight so easily?"

Suppose you had a broken leg and your doctor treated it simply with a shot of painkiller and sent you home. When the painkiller wore off, you would realize the doctor hadn't treated the basic problem. He should have set your leg in a cast. Well, that is what we do when we diet away our fat. When we finish a diet, we may have lost some fat but our tendency to get fat is still there. The problem is that something inside is making us gain weight faster than other people do. Something in our body chemistry is favoring the deposit of fat.

When a naturally skinny persons eats 1000 calories, all of them get burned, wasted, or somehow used up. When a fat person eats 1000 calories, perhaps only 900 of them are used up and the remaining 100 are converted to fat. For years, nutritionists have explained this with the observation that fat people exercise less. Well, that isn't the whole story. The fat person's body adjusts somehow to the making of excess fat.

Our conclusion has to be: Yes, people who have gotten too fat may need to go on a diet to get the fat off. Once most of the excess fat is off, however, they are really only at the beginning of their treatment. At that point they must tackle the real problem. How can they change their body chemistries so that they won't have such a tendency to make fat out of the foods they eat? How can they avoid getting fat all over again? There is a way that we can alter every person's chemistry so that fewer calories are converted to fat. We can't make the superfat into superskinnys, but we can improve everyone a little.

3

The Body Machine

FOR YEARS there has been one standard answer for overweight people; either you eat too much, exercise too little, or both. Doctors, nutritionists, and dieticians all echo the "party line." Well, it simply isn't true! There are people who get fat easily and people who remain skin and bones no matter how much they eat or how little they exercise. Not only can two people differ radically in their tendency to get fat, but also the same person can change radically in his lifetime. Women who decide to take birth control pills often gain more easily. The "party line" would be that they started to eat more or exercise less, but thousands of women claim the contrary.

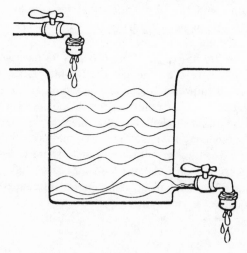

Figure 1

The traditional approach to overweight is often pictured by a diagram of a water tank (Figure 1). Water is added to the tank by a faucet above and water is let out of the tank by a faucet below. Humans are supposed to be just like this tank. Increasing the flow from the upper faucet is like eating more calories, and the level in the tank goes up. The lower faucet is supposed to be similar to exercise, so that closing the faucet is like decreasing your daily exercise and the level of fat in your body goes up. Well, this analogy is partly true; getting fat is largely a matter of eating too much and exercising too little. Unfortunately, the analogy breaks down under practical everyday experience because it implies that people are passive reservoirs, affected only by outside food supply and exercise. The fact is we are not passive reservoirs or tanks, but active metabolizing machines, each different, each handling calories differently. I prefer to think of the body as a machine that runs efficiently or inefficiently, depending on circumstances. Just as an automobile may be tuned up properly and get more mileage from its fuel, the human machine is also subject to change.

Most people are unaware that 60–70 percent of the energy that muscles need when one is resting is supplied by fat. That is, fats, either from a recent meal or from fat deposits, travel through the blood to muscle, where they contribute more than half of the resting muscle's energy needs. Glucose and fats are burned side by side all day long, but fats supply most of the energy.

Storage of fat is therefore a natural body function. The trouble is that fat people are overly proficient at storing fat and have less than normal proficiency at burning it.

Our analogy with the tank of water doesn't hold completely because some people's body machines work harder to store fat than other people's. It isn't simply a matter of "You eat too much or you exercise too little."

Furthermore, unlike the analogy with the water tank, being fat tends to make you get even fatter. Fatness is a vicious cycle; the more fat you have, the more your body chemistry, or metabolism, changes to favor the build-up of even more fat.

4

Fat Floats!

IF YOU THROW a pound of butter in a swimming pool, it will float just like a cork. When oil tankers collide at sea, they spill oil, a form of fat, which floats on top of the ocean. The fat in your body is no different. The more fat you've got, the better you will be able to float in a swimming pool. When I was a boy, I had a girlfriend who could float so well that she could read a book while lying calmly on top of the water. One day she asked why I never floated. Naturally I told her I could float if I wanted to, I just didn't want to. Well, the truth is, when she finally got me to try, I sank like a rock. It made me mad and I vowed that I would some-day be able to perform this marvelous feat just as well as she. Well, that's just what happened . . . I got fat.

In contrast to fat, lean muscle and bone do not float. Scientists call that part of the body the Lean Body Mass. It is quite prac-tical to think of the body as having two distinct parts, the fat part that floats and the Lean Body Mass that sinks. There are many

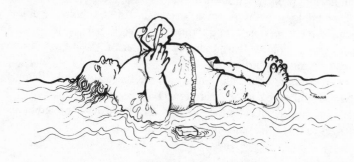

Fat Floats!

ways to estimate the amount of body fat but by far the most precise method is based on how well one floats. A large water tank is used in which one can be completely immersed while sitting on a pipe frame chair hung from a scale. The scale with its hanging chair looks much like the scale in the vegetable section of the supermarket. The more bone and muscle you have, the more easily you sink and the more you weigh under water. The more fat you have, the more you tend to float and the less you weigh under water. Big fat people approaching our water tank are afraid they might break our scale. But the truth is, the fatter they are, the lighter they are under water. Under water, it's the skinny people who weigh the most. It sounds funny, but we compliment people who are very dense. To us, dense is beautiful.

The underwater immersion test is the most accurate method for body fat determination, and many universities use it in their physical fitness education programs. It involves some sophisticated equipment, so one can't easily do it in his backyard swimming pool. But there is a game that you can try in a swimming pool, based on the same principle, that will give you an approximation of your fat level. Get two or more people to float on their backs after having filled their lungs with air. Then when someone signals, "Go!," everyone blows his air out. Slowly, everyone should begin to sink. The one to hit bottom first is the leanest.

Above 25 percent fat, people float easily.

At 22–23 percent fat (healthy for a woman), one can usually float while breathing shallowly.

At 15 percent fat (low for a woman, healthy for a man), one will usually sink very slowly even with a full chest of air.

At 13 percent fat, one will sink readily even with a full chest of air, even in salty ocean water.

These numbers are only approximates because one's floatability is also affected by age, lung volume, and water temperature. Underwater weighing isn't as simple as it sounds and can't be done accurately as a backyard operation.

I once did this test with a very lean marathon runner, Carl. As I slowly settled on the bottom of the pool, I looked over at Carl. He had hit the bottom so hard that he had bounced up and was coming down a second time!

While there are many other techniques for determination of body fat, most are based only on subcutaneous fat that can be seen and pinched. They are much less accurate because they don't take into account the hidden intramuscular fat. Even worse, they give no estimate of Lean Body Mass. The water tank method allows us to measure small changes in the amount of body muscle as well as changes in body fat.

Authorities disagree somewhat, but I think it is safe to say that 15 percent fat for men and 22 percent fat for women are maximums for good health. Good athletes often have much less. Thin, cross-country runners often are as low as 6 percent. Professional football teams have been measured, with the heavyweight linemen averaging about 17 percent and the faster-moving quarterbacks averaging about 13 percent. The linemen, you notice, are a little over our theoretical 15 percent because a little extra fat means extra weight and is presumably an advantage. But we question whether this is conducive to good health since these are the men who "turn to fat" the quickest when they give up the sport.

The greater fat level for women, even when normal and healthy, may partially account for the greater incidence of obesity in women than men. Since women have more fat to start with, it's probably easier for them to get even fatter.

These percentages, 15 percent for men and 22 percent for women, are the highest maximum percentages that one can have and still be considered in the range of normal. We have measured thousands of people, however, and most men seem to average 23 percent fat, most women 36 percent. Don't confuse *average* with *normal.* To be 5 or 10 pounds overweight may be *average,* and all your friends may be the same, but that doesn't mean you're *normal.*

At this point, the question of body type often arises. One probably reasons that 15 percent and 22 percent are normals for mesomorphs, but shouldn't ectomorphs, the "naturally skinnys," be less than that? And shouldn't the endomorphs, the "naturally fatsos," be more? My answer is an emphatic no! All men should strive for 15 percent maximum fat. If a man has large bones and much muscle, he can carry more fat without exceeding the 15 percent. His total weight can be greater than another man of the same height who has slender bones, but they should both shoot for 15 percent fat or less.

I have seen many people who would have been called "naturally fatsos," or endomorphs, but who have subsequently brought their fat level down to a point where they don't fit the endomorph label anymore. It is even more astonishing to see the high content of fat in many ectomorphs who appear quite thin, even skinny.

Rather than use these words to describe apparent differences in body type, I prefer to discard them completely in favor of fat percentages.

5

Overweight versus Overfat

MOST PEOPLE are concerned if they are overweight, but the term is obsolete. We have known all along that overweight people were overweight because they had excess fat. But now we realize that fat can be hidden inside the body in such a way that you can be carrying a lot of excess fat without seeming overweight at all. Take, for example, the former weight lifter. Once he was very strong, with lean, hard muscles. Since giving up the heavy physical stuff, his muscles have turned to fat somewhat. He may be the same weight now as before, but now it's fat weight instead of muscle weight. He has become overfat without getting overweight.

The sad thing is that the same process has taken place in 90 percent of adult Americans. Up to the age of fifteen, the majority of us are very active, using calories as fast as we eat them. But then we "grow up." We settle down to the adult activities of drinking, working, and commuting in cars. Our muscles gradually become less dense, less lean, and more fatty.

A similar scene can be visualized with beef cattle raised on the range. Young heifers romp and cavort, stopping only occasionally to nurse from their mothers. Gradually they settle down and their wonderfully lean muscles go to fat. With lack of hard use, the muscles develop those streaks of fat we call marbling. The more streaking (or marbling) of fat in the muscles, the more we prize the muscles as steaks.

Just as with beef cattle, humans become less active as they mature. Most of my adult patients mistakenly believe they are just as active, or perhaps even more active, as adults than they were as kids. But they are confusing the meaning of physical activity. I am talking about sports activities that really put muscles to work, that really stress muscles to capacity from time to time. Don't think of a long day's work cleaning house, cooking meals, picking up after kids, or on your feet at any job as real muscular activity. Such work may leave you exhausted at the end of the day, but to your muscles, it is only busywork. Such routine daily work may never amount to more than 50 percent stress to your muscle and hence 50 percent of your muscle can atrophy, to be replaced by fat. Don't confuse work with exercise.

As your muscles turn to fat, you may not be gaining weight because fat is merely replacing unused muscle. Most adults who weigh the same at forty as they did at twenty have nevertheless gotten very fat. We start to gain weight only when we have so excessively overeaten and underexercised that we exceed the capacity of the muscles to get internally fat. Then the fat begins to deposit outside the muscles under the skin. This fat is no longer replacing muscle but is adding to the body, and you get overweight. People who are just starting to get overweight are usually already overfat. If you are only 5 pounds *overweight,* it is probable that you are at least 13 pounds *overfat.*

To emphasize in another way the difference between being heavy and being fat, let me tell you a true story about a 285-pound football player. He was a valuable man on one of the big West Coast pro football teams but each month his coach fined him for being overweight. He was only 5 feet 10 inches tall, so his coach reasoned that he would have to be fat to weigh so much for that height. This went on for a year or more, with the big man dieting all the time, unsuccessfully trying to meet his coach's idea of ideal weight. Finally one of the universities engaged in research on fat and physical performance agreed to determine the percentage of body fat of each player on the football team. To the amazement of all, our 285-pound man came out 2 percent fat, an astonishingly low number considering that 15 percent fat for men is considered normal. Needless to say, his coach stopped fining him, and he stopped his starvation dieting. He gained weight to 325 pounds, a more normal fat content for him, felt much stronger, and performed much better on the football field.

Here then is a case of confusing weight with fat. You can make no realistic determination of how fat you are by your weight.

My own life provides another example of the confusion between overweight and overfat. My case is the opposite of the football player's, and more typical of American fatsos. It also illustrates the worthlessness of the bathroom scales that we rely on so much. For the majority of my life, I have not fluctuated in weight. From the age of twenty to thirty-seven, I was 170 pounds with less than ½ pound change. I was one of those obnoxious people who eats anything and everything without the slightest change in weight. So, when I started to gain weight rapidly at the age of thirty-seven, I was startled and looked hard for a cause for the change. Since my weight had been so steady for so long, it seemed obvious that I must have made some rather radical change in my life as I turned thirty-seven. Though I searched my own memory and questioned my friends, I could not discover any significant change at that time of my life. I considered possible emotional conflict, troubles at work, sickness, medications, smoking — everything. There was nothing I could put my finger on.

Then it occurred to me that perhaps a significant change had taken place a long time previously that hadn't hatched into a weight problem until I turned thirty-seven. And there was the answer! At thirty-two, I had had a most radical change in life style. I got a job. And with the job, I had money. I had huge business lunches, each with two or three drinks. At the same time, I gave up all the extremely active sports life that had been my way before. You have to picture this — a trim thirty-two-year-old man, drastically increasing his daily calories, including rich foods and alcohol, and at the same time equally drastically reducing his calorie expenditure. He would have to get fat, right? The "party line" says he would have to get fat. Well, *I didn't gain a pound for nearly five years*. So I thought I wasn't getting fat. In fact, I used to gloat in front of my business associates. Clearly, God intended that I would be eternally beautifully thin. And Then It Happened! I started gaining weight like everybody else.

From previous chapters it should be clear that I was really getting fat from the day of the big change when I turned thirty-two. But for nearly five years, the fat went into my muscles as the muscle itself atrophied from disuse. In other words, the fat replaced the muscle. With one thing merely replacing the other, I didn't gain any weight. I was getting fatter but not heavier. But muscles can only hold just so much fat! In due time muscular degeneration slows and calories deposit outside the muscle, under the skin. This subcutaneous fat is not replacing anything; it is simply an addition. So I gained weight. I got fat for five years before I started gaining weight.

6

What Is Your Correct Weight?

IN CALCULATING your correct weight, we start with your Lean Body Mass. We can't start with the size of your bones, the width of your shoulders, your age, your height, or your body type. The weight tables that your physician uses are based on several of these factors put together. Such tables were useful when nothing better was available but it is clear now that they can be off by 20–30 pounds for any individual. It is possible to be overweight according to the charts and yet be underfat. And the reverse is true. We have measured many skinny people who are underweight according to the charts but are overfat. They have no visible subcutaneous fat but their muscles are loaded with intramuscular fat.

We determine a person's ideal weight by the size of his frame, or Lean Body Mass. If you have large bones and muscles, we would project a greater weight for you than for someone else of your same height who has thin bones.

Figure 2. Male at 15% fat

Total Weight	Fat	LBM	Age	Activity
170 lbs.	25 lbs.	145 lbs.	20	Wrestling
162 lbs.	24 lbs.	138 lbs.	38	Running
135 lbs.	20 lbs.	115 lbs.	45	Prison camp

Male maintaining 15% body fat despite decreasing muscle mass as activities change.

Let's take an example of a man at three different occasions in his life (Figure 2). First he is twenty years old and into college wrestling, gymnastics, and weight lifting. All three activities have added muscle to his frame so that his Lean Body Mass (LBM) is

145 pounds. He can carry 25 pounds of fat and weigh 170 pounds.

At the age of thirty-eight, he is a businessman whose only real physical activity beyond weekend skiing and some golf is jogging. The jogging keeps him lean and healthy but is not a sport that "packs on" much muscle. In fact, in a case like this the jogging will actually decrease some of his upper body muscle! So now he has only 138 pounds of Lean Body Mass. Now he shouldn't carry over 24 pounds of fat and shouldn't exceed 162 pounds. His body adapts beautifully to its new role. Obviously, a runner doesn't need the upper body musculature of a gymnast. As the muscle mass decreases, the total weight should decrease also.

Let's take a third case. Suppose our man, now in his forties, undergoes some extreme deprivation, such as two years of near starvation in a prison camp or perhaps a chronic debilitating disease for several years. He will lose much fat and much muscle. At the end of such hardship, he will be haggard and thin. His mother and probably his physician will want to fatten him up. I emphatically disagree. If his lean mass has dropped to 115 pounds, he should not carry over 20 pounds of fat and shouldn't weigh more than 135. The only healthy recourse for such an individual is to replace the lost muscle, adding fat only to maintain 15 percent. If he eats to add weight, he will only add fat weight and will end up obese, just like the more typical fatso — even though he may still appear thin.

Most sedentary Americans not only show a decrease in lean mass as they grow older but also an increase in fat content.

Consider the changes in a sedentary woman. Let's say that at age twenty she is a healthy 22 percent fat and weighs 120 pounds. By age thirty-five she is proud that she has gained only 5 pounds but it would be quite typical for her to be 30 percent fat. If you look at the table in Figure 3, you will see that she has actually

Figure 3. Typical Body Composition Changes in a Sedentary Woman

Age	%Fat	Total Weight	Fat	LBM	Ideal Max. Weight
20	22%	120 lbs.	26 lbs.	94 lbs.	120 lbs.
35	30%	125 lbs.	38 lbs.	87 lbs.	112 lbs.

gained 12 pounds of fat while losing 7 pounds of muscle. Her Lean Body Mass is now only 87 pounds, and to be 22 percent fat, she should not weigh more than 112.

You can see that the term "correct weight" is really quite ambiguous. A person's "correct weight" changes as his lean mass changes. If our sample woman exercises, she can rebuild her lean mass to the former 94 pounds and, in a sense, earn the right to weigh 120 pounds again. If she won't exercise, her correct weight is 112 pounds.

Incidentally, the amount of Lean Body Mass one has also largely determines how much one should eat. After all, it's the Lean Body Mass that burns up the calories we eat. When you put gas in your car, it's the size engine that determines the gas consumption, not the size of the car. For all practical purposes the fat part doesn't need calories. You don't need to feed calories to your fat; fat *is* calories. Two people may weigh the same amount and yet one may have more fat, and therefore less Lean Body Mass, than the other. If they both eat the same number of calories, the one with the smaller Lean Body Mass will gain weight. In the next few years, calorie charts will become available that will tell you how many calories you can eat, based on your pounds of Lean Body Mass.

In calculating ideal maximum weight, we have to start with what is real, the part of you that functions, that all day burns calories, even when you are asleep. We have to start with the amount of active metabolizing tissue you have, your Lean Body Mass. Then we calculate how many pounds of fat we could add to your Lean Body Mass so that you would then be 22 percent fat (or 15 percent for men). If you would exercise in such a way that your Lean Body Mass would increase, your need for calories would increase, and you could carry more fat without exceeding the ideal 22 percent (15 percent for men).

7

What Is the Cure for All This Fat?

THE FIRST THING is to get it firmly in your head that it isn't the excess fat that is so bad; it's the lack of athletically trained muscle that is at the root of it all. Carrying an extra 20 pounds of fat isn't as bad as we have been told. Suppose you carried around a 20-pound knapsack all day. Would that be bad? The extra load might be a strain on someone in poor physical condition, but if the weight were added slowly it might actually be a good way to get in shape. When I was on the ski patrol, skiing all day with 10 pounds of first aid equipment didn't bother me at all. A few years later, when I was 10 pounds *overweight,* I really noticed it. The point here is not to prove that extra fat is good but to show that it's the lack of good muscle that is bad. It's the underlying body changes accompanying the extra fat that do you in.

As muscle turns to fat, not only does the actual quantity of muscle decrease, thereby decreasing the need for calories, but also the chemistry of the remaining muscle changes in such a way as to use fewer calories.

Dieting may decrease the weight of your knapsack of fat, but it cannot increase the amount of muscle nor reverse the badly altered chemistry of the muscles. Dieting attacks subcutaneous fat first and will remove intramuscular fat only under the most severe prison camp circumstances. Even if you were willing to undergo such rigor, the results would be disappointing because you still have done nothing to prevent yourself from getting fat all over again. Furthermore, you may have actually worsened your situation, because radical dieting, unbalanced dieting, shots, and fasting have been shown to lessen muscle mass while you are losing fat. In fact, there is good evidence now that one should get fit first *before* embarking on any kind of diet program. A well-exercised body seems to respond more quickly and with less muscle loss to the stress of dieting.

We have developed such a mania for losing weight that we overlook what the lost weight may consist of.

Suppose I were to call you on the telephone with the exciting news that the local supermarket was selling twelve pounds for only $1.29! Your reaction would be, "Twelve pounds of what?" Well, that's my reaction when someone tells me of a terrific diet which guarantees that you can lose twelve pounds in no time at all — twelve pounds of what?

There are nationally known weight-watching organizations in which a loss of weight is the only criterion of a member's success. Unfortunately, while losing fat, the member may also be losing muscle, which decreases the need for calories and augments the problem. All of us can think of friends who have gone on diets only to end up looking gaunt and haggard. We admonish them and tell them they really would look better with a little fat on them. But it isn't the loss of fat that gives them a wasted appearance. It's the muscle loss! Additionally, a muscle and fat loss due to dieting does nothing to improve body shape. If the person was fat and pear-shaped before a radical diet, he'll end up skinny and pear-shaped after.

Earlier I mentioned that many people who appear skinny are sometimes high in fat. They have done what most people do when they want to gain weight. They eat. And when one overeats to gain weight the added weight is only *fat* weight. The skinny person doesn't really look more shapely with a gain in fat weight. He or she usually loses the waistline, the shoulders narrow a little more, the thighs and buttocks fatten up, and a double chin may even develop. In other words, overeating to gain weight will only add fat and will put it in places where you need it the least.

Compare these overeaters and undereaters to the many people who have exercised their bodies into low fat levels. They are full-bodied, healthy individuals who can lead active lives without a constant concern for the number of calories they eat.

Exercise increases muscle, tones it, alters its chemistry, and increases its metabolic rate. All of these cause you to burn more calories even when asleep.

The ultimate cure for obesity is exercise!

The most efficient exercises for this purpose are called aerobics. Briefly, aerobic exercise means steady exercise, exercise that demands an uninterrupted output from your muscles over a 12-minute period. It has been shown in many exercise physiology laboratories that a steady continuous exercise repeated every day reverses more quickly the syndrome of muscle turning to fat than any other kind. In other words, if we want to make muscle lean again while removing the marbled fat, we must replace the fat with lean muscle. This does not mean making big, bulky muscle such as the weight lifter wants. It does mean making lean again the muscle you already have. Most people don't want to do body building in the sense of weight lifting; they want the muscle they already have to be lean and functional. Steady, endurance kind of muscular work does just that. As the muscle gets leaner, metabolism changes automatically, and you burn more calories without even knowing it.

The word aerobic means air, but more specifically refers to the oxygen in the air. The muscles need oxygen to function and their need for oxygen goes up dramatically when we work them. We can measure how hard a muscle is working by how much oxygen it is using (or burning). As you exercise harder, you need more oxygen, and the heart rate goes up. Increases in your heart rate due to exercise are an indirect measure of how hard your muscles are working.

If you make a muscle work too hard, its need for oxygen will be greater than your heart and blood can deliver. Aerobic exercises make the muscles work hard enough to need lots of oxygen but not so hard as to exceed the ability of the heart and blood to deliver it.

Exercise such as this, hard but not too hard, and continuous for a minimum of 12 minutes, does more to tone or firm up the muscles than other kinds of exercise. All I am really saying is that aerobic exercise is the *most efficient* way to remove the marbling fat, which in turn is the most efficient way to change your metabolism so you won't get fat anymore. Anything we do that uses our muscles could be called exercise. And any exercise, even the household chores I made fun of earlier, helps to keep muscle intact. But to retain a full complement of muscle, we need exercise that uses it fully. Most people are limited in the time they can spend on an exercise program and some would prefer not to exercise at all. So, the shortest exercise of greatest efficiency should have wide appeal.

You can get as much benefit from 15 minutes of jogging as from 2 hours of tennis. You might make your muscles perfectly lean by playing tennis but you will have to play hard, 2–3 hours a day, six to seven days a week. For most people, it would be much better to do a steady 12-minute aerobic exercise every day for fat control and conditioning, and then play tennis for fun!

The main criterion of aerobic exercise is that it be continuous and steady. We don't know exactly why it works, but it does. There is something about pushing a muscle to work hard at a steady pace that leads quickly to a firming of the muscle and a loss of its marbling. Stop-and-go exercises just don't do the same thing as quickly. There are very strong weight lifters who cannot run a mile and whose muscles are loaded with fat. These are people who "go to fat" if they become inactive.

Figure 4 contains a list of steady endurance exercises that fit the aerobic definition, compared with a list of nonaerobic exercises that are either too "stop and go," too short in duration, or of too low an intensity.

Figure 4

AEROBIC	NONAEROBIC		
	Stop and Go	Short Duration	Low Intensity
Running/Jogging	Tennis	Weight Lifting	Golf
Cross-Country Skiing	Downhill Skiing	Sprinting	Canasta
Jumping Rope	Football	Isometrics	
Running in Place	Calisthenics	Square Dancing	
Cycling Outdoors	Handball		
Stationary Bicycle	Racquetball		
Rowing			
Mini-trampoline			

There seems to be something magical about doing 12 minutes of an aerobic exercise. In fact, we can't even classify an exercise as aerobic unless it lasts for a minimum of 12 minutes — nonstop. Two 6-minute exercises don't add up to one 12-minute exercise. I don't mean that 6-minute exercises are worthless; I mean that they are less efficient at producing the heart and muscle enzyme changes that are so valuable in altering our metabolism. Twelve minutes is the *minimum* recommended time for any exercise. Some exercises require more time to achieve the same effect because during the first few minutes, the heart rate hasn't reached the training rate. (Training rate will be discussed in Chapter 8.)

In Figure 5 several of the best aerobic exercises have been separated into three categories based on this principle. If you choose an exercise from Category II, which has a 15-minute minimum

Figure 5. Aerobic Exercises

I Required Minimum Time 12 Minutes	II Required Minimum Time 15 Minutes	III Required Minimum Time 20 Minutes
Jumping Rope Running in Place Jumping Jacks Chair Stepping	Jogging Running Cross-Country Skiing Rowing Dancing Mini-trampoline	Walking Outdoor Bicycling Stationary Bicycling Ice Skating Roller Skating Swimming

time, it will take your heart about three minutes to reach your training rate. If you choose an exercise from Category III, it will take about eight minutes to reach your training rate. In effect, one must tack on "warm-up" time to the 12 minutes of exercise.

If you find that when you run (a Category II exercise), it takes only one minute for your heart to reach its training rate, theoretically you could finish your exercise in 13 minutes. I advise against this, however. Do not try to "warm up" fast by running fast in the first few minutes. Conversely, if it takes your heart a longer time to reach the training rate, then you must exercise longer than the suggested time. The rule is, exercise 12 minutes at your training rate plus however long it takes your heart to reach that training rate. It is difficult to determine this on your own, so I urge you just to stick to the chart.

The next logical question is, if 12 minutes at the training heart rate is good, wouldn't 24 minutes be better? The answer is definitely yes. But the first 12 minutes produce a much more lasting effect than the second 12 minutes. We urge people to exercise longer than 12 minutes if they wish, knowing that their improvement will be faster. We must admit, however, that you get less and less for your effort beyond the 12-minute point. It's another application of the law of diminishing returns. It is for this reason that we urge the 12-minute exercise six days a week rather than a 30-minute exercise three days a week. People who are already quite fit may profit more from the latter. For them, extra long exercise may be the only way to reach a competition training level. But we don't suggest this for the other ninety-eight percent of the population.

What about warming up and cooling down? In general, these should both be a "dress rehearsal" of your exercise. If you decide to jog, then the best warm-up is a very slow jog. And the best cool-down is a fast walk. The same would be true of all the exercises. Just do a slower version of the exercise to warm up or cool down. For most people 3–5 minutes is sufficient time for warming up or cooling down.

Some people are stiff when they first start to exercise. A few minutes of simple stretches should relieve this. Touch your toes, stretch your arms overhead, and bend at the waist from side to side. But, *please,* do these stretches *slowly.* If they're done too fast and vigorously, the muscle reacts in a manner exactly the opposite of what you want. It cramps up and leaves you very sore.

Please don't misinterpret my emphasis on exercise. I do *not* mean that each daily exercise burns up lots of calories. Jogging for 20 minutes, for example, consumes only 180 calories, approximately the caloric content of a glass of milk. You would have to jog for days to use up the calories in a hot fudge sundae. There are many studies in the literature that support the point that each minute of exercise uses few calories. But we use calories when we are *not* exercising, even when we are asleep; and the exercised body seems to do more of this.

Furthermore, such studies overlook the long-term cumulative effects. It is ridiculous to expect reversal of muscle enzyme loss and of fatty muscle infiltration in such short periods. Such changes take many months or even years in very fat people.

The point of this chapter is that proper exercise changes muscle, which in turn alters body use of calories. It is a simple fact that those who exercise aerobically on a regular schedule do not get fat. If I were offering a pill to decrease the tendency of the body to make fat, fat people would be lining up to buy it. I *am* offering such a pill; it takes just 12 minutes a day to swallow it!

8

How Hard Should I Exercise?

THE ANSWER to the above question is based on efficiency. Let's say you pick jogging as your exercise. If you jog too slowly, it may take forever to get the desired effect; if you jog too fast, you just wear yourself out and get nowhere. Obviously, there is an in-between point at which you are working your muscles hard enough for maximum benefit but not overdoing it. Since it's hard to measure the muscle activity itself, we measure the oxygen demand of the muscles. As the oxygen demand goes up, your heart beats faster. As you exercise harder and harder, your heart rate goes faster and faster.

As indicated in Figure 6, your heart rate reaches a maximum for your age at which it cannot beat any faster no matter how much harder you exercise. For young people, twenty years or less, this maximum is about 200 beats a minute. A forty-year-old person's heart has an absolute maximum of 180 beats a minute.

You would think that a well-trained athlete would have a higher maximum pulse than someone who isn't physically fit. Not so. You'd also think that women would have higher maximum pulses than men since they are generally smaller animals. But again, there are only slight differences between men's and women's maximum pulses. In fact, the only thing that affects the maximum pulse is age. The older you are, the slower your heart beats during maximum exercise.

These maximum heart rates for different ages should be practiced only by athletes during maximum athletic competition. For regular, everyday, efficient exercise we should work only hard enough to make our hearts go at 80 percent of the maximum for our age. If you are forty, your maximum heart rate is 182, and

Figure 6. Recommended Heart Rates During Exercise

Age	Maximum Heart Rate	85% of Max. (Athlete-Training Rate)	80% of Max. (Recommended Training Rate)	75% of Max. (Heart Disease History)
				Not to exceed
20	200	170	160	150
22	198	168	158	148
24	196	167	157	147
26	194	165	155	145
28	192	163	154	144
30	190	162	152	143
32	189	161	151	142
34	187	159	150	140
36	186	158	149	140
38	184	156	147	138
40	182	155	146	137
45	179	152	143	134
50	175	149	140	131
55	171	145	137	128
60	160	136	128	120
65+	150	128	120	113

Based on resting heart rates of 72 for males and 80 for females. Men over forty and people with **any** heart problem should have a stress electrocardiogram before starting an exercise program.

you should exercise hard enough to get your heart going 80 percent of that maximum 182. 80 percent of 182 equals 146 beats per minute.

Let's consider three forty-year-old men. The first is terribly out of shape, which means he has a lot of intramuscular fat as well as some obvious subcutaneous fat bulging under his skin. He might easily drive his pulse to 146 by just walking briskly. A second man, in better shape, might have to jog to get 146 beats per minute. And a third forty-year-old, lean and athletic, might have to run quite a fast pace to reach the same heart rate. It might appear that the third man is getting the most exercise, while the first man is being quite lazy. But in fact, they are all exercising equally, getting the same heart, lung, and muscular benefits.

For years the fat man who has tried to jog with his trim friend has felt he must jog at the same speed to get the same exercise.

Now you can see that you should walk, jog, or run at whatever speed gives you the correct heart beat.

Husbands who are athletic are particularly guilty of pushing their wives into too strenuous exercise. They coerce their wives into going out for "just a little jog together." He runs slower for her and she runs faster for him. One is underexercised, the other is overexercised, and it is inefficient exercise for both of them. Men and women should think twice about exercising together because of their differences in muscle mass. The average man has 20 percent more muscle than the average woman, and he has 30 percent less fat.

Women, don't let this discourage you. While men may be stronger in exercises that demand a lot of power, there is growing evidence that women are better endowed for endurance activities. Exercise by yourself or with another woman and you'll enjoy it more. The only time men and women should run together is if the man is several years older than the woman, or if he is quite out of condition and the woman is in good condition.

Never again let anyone push you into exercising at his rate. Just take a look at the heart rate table in Figure 6 to determine the correct exercise heart rate for you. Then pick any one of the steady aerobic exercises listed, or for that matter, any steady exercise. Do that exercise, at that heart rate, for at least 12 minutes nonstop six days per week. The first few times you should stop after a minute or two to take your pulse. Count your pulse with a sweep-second hand for 6 seconds and multiply by ten to get beats per minute. (More on this in Chapter 10.) If the pulse is less than your correct exercise heart rate, you aren't exercising hard enough. If the pulse is too high, just slow down a bit. Taking your own pulse like this is called "pulse-monitored exercise." It's as if you were being watched over by the world's best coach.

I'm asked repeatedly if older people, or people who are badly out of shape should "ease" into an exercise program. Isn't it too much for such people to start right out at 12 minutes a day? Certainly not! The whole point of pulse-monitored exercise is that it prevents one from overexercising. If you are terribly out of shape, you may not even be able to walk briskly for the required period without undue stress. I don't care if you have to crawl — do it for a full 12 minutes. You can use 70 percent maximum heart rate for a few weeks if you wish and then move up to 80 percent. You can increase the intensity gradually but you should do a sustained exercise right from the beginning.

It's the time you spend urging your body to change that really matters. The body adapts beautifully to steady pressure just as teeth can be moved by the gentle steady pressure of braces. I see men running like crazy around the local track, proud that they can cover a mile or so in 6 minutes flat and then wondering why they still must fight a bulging waistline. Such exertions are as effective in weight control as trying to move teeth with a hammer. Run slower and longer and let your body adjust.

The heart rate table assumes that your average heart rate at rest is near the average of 72 beats per minute for men and 80 for women. When a person's resting heart rate is very low, it is excessive exercise to push the heart rate up to the number on the table. If your resting heart rate is 12 beats per minute, or more, below average, we suggest you revise your exercise heart rate downward by applying a formula:

(Maximum — Resting) × 65 percent + Resting = Training Heart Rate

Let's work through an example: Your average resting heart rate is 55 and you are forty years old. Maximum for a forty year old is 182. 182 minus 55 equals 127. 65 percent of 127 equals 82.5. 82.5 plus 55 equals 137.5. Your exercise heart rate should be 137–138 rather than 146 as shown in the table.

One urgent caution! Look at the column labeled 75 percent of maximum. It's sad indeed, to read a book like this and get charged up with enthusiasm, only to exercise yourself into a heart attack. All physiologists, physicians, and heart specialists agree that *proper* exercise is beneficial even for people with bad hearts. The trouble comes in defining the word *proper*. The 75 percent maximum column is being used by physicians in treatment of heart patients all over the world. But! If you have any history of heart ailment, by all means be cleared for such a program by a physician before you start.

Heart attacks are so common in the United States and so disastrous that I can't pass up the chance for a few comments. There is no longer any question that regular aerobic exercise is a deterrent to heart attack. But there are also cases of people dropping dead of a heart attack while jogging, and they were jogging so they wouldn't have a heart attack! A few doctors use these isolated cases of heart attack during exercise as a reason for discouraging exercise. That's like saying we should do away with ambulances because they may have a wreck on the way to the hospital.

Still, people do have heart attacks while exercising, particularly if they neglect to check their heart rates as suggested in this chapter. The best way to find out if you are potentially one of these people is to have a stress electrocardiogram (EKG). (Most EKGs are taken with the person lying down and hence are no measure of possible abnormality during exercise. Such tests are called resting EKGs.) To find out how the heart will function during exercise, the patient is asked to walk, then jog, and then run on a treadmill while the heart is being monitored by an EKG machine. This is called a stress EKG and will reliably indicate the possibility of a heart attack during exercise. Furthermore, the speed of the treadmill is increased gradually so the intensity of the effort by the patient can be increased gradually. The physician can stop the test at the first sign of abnormality rather than waiting for a heart attack.

Your car may run perfectly when it's idling but run poorly at high speed on the highway. So your mechanic has to race the engine during tune-ups to get an idea of how it's going to function at highway speeds. Similarly, if your doctor gives you a "complete" physical exam, including urinalysis, blood chemistry, and a resting EKG, and finds nothing wrong, all he can really say is, "You will be fine, as long as you don't move."

The stress EKG is an excellent test to have before starting on an exercise program, particularly for men over forty and others in the high-risk group. Unfortunately, stress EKGs are expensive. Many people hesitate at the price, and even some with occasional chest pain indicative of heart disease will exercise without a stress EKG. If you are one of these, I implore you, beg you, to pulse-monitor your exercise, using the 6-second pulse technique and the proper exercise heart rate for you. I give many lectures on this subject around the country and sometimes, when it's possible, I get the audience to go outside with me after my talk to practice the

techniques. I stand in one place and have people jog to a desig-
nated tree or post and back to me. We take pulses immediately
upon their return. About 70 percent of the time the pulse will be
too high, indicating that the individual went too fast. So I send that
person off to try again at a slower pace and the pulse is often still
too high. By the third or fourth try, people are saying, "I had no
idea how slowly you wanted me to run." Many of them realize
that they can't run or jog at all; that they can maintain 80 percent
maximum heart rate by walking fast.

Aerobic Exercises

A. Steady, Nonstop

B. Duration — 12 Minutes Minimum

C. Intensity — 80% of Maximum Heart Rate

9

If Two Aspirins Are Good,
Four Must Be Better

NOTICE THAT the heart rate table, Figure 6, also contains an 85 percent column. Trained athletes, familiar with competition, can benefit from exercise of greater intensity. They should exercise at 85 percent of their maximums. Please don't make the mistake of putting yourself in this column if you don't belong there. Men in particular are inclined to do this on the grounds that if moderate exercise is good, intense exercise is better. If your body isn't ready for it, you will overheat the muscles, doing more damage than good. If you want fast improvement, you should exercise longer rather than harder.

When Hal walked into my clinic after a six-month absence, my jaw dropped. The man looked five years older and sick! I managed to hide my dismay because Hal was obviously elated. "I've lost 20 pounds in six months just from running," he said proudly. And it was true, Hal was thinner — to the point of gauntness. Something was seriously wrong. Sure enough, when he was tested for body fat, he had lost both fat *and* muscle!

Of the 20 pounds he had lost, 7½ were muscle. (See Figure 7.) That explained why he looked so hollow, his skin seemed to hang. I thought for sure Hal had gone on some strange diet but, when questioned, he insisted that it was only the running that had caused him to lose weight. Then it hit me! Hal must have been *over*exercising. Not only will you lose muscle if you diet improperly, you will also lose muscle if you overexercise!

And that is what had happened. Hal had decided that he wanted to get in shape really fast, so every day for six months, he had run

Figure 7. Loss of Lean Mass Due to Overexercise

Hal	Before	After
Total Weight	170 lbs.	150 lbs.
% Fat	25%	20%
LBM	127.5 lbs.	120 lbs.
Fat	42.5 lbs.	30 lbs.

two miles with a heart rate of 160 beats per minute. This was a reasonable heart rate if Hal had been twenty years old, but Hal was fifty. Every day for six months he had been driving his heart rate nearly 15 percent over the recommended rate. This was overstressing his muscles and they weren't able to repair themselves.

Hal was overexercising in a second way. He was exercising too often with the same exercise. After the age of forty, you should switch exercises from day to day. (For example, run on Monday, Wednesday, and Friday, and cycle on Tuesday, Thursday, and Saturday.) The reason is that muscles can't repair as quickly when you get older. By switching exercises, you give the set of muscles you stressed on Monday time to build up while you stress another set on Tuesday. By Wednesday, the "Monday muscles" are not only repaired but also stronger than ever.

So poor Hal had put his muscles in double jeopardy. They were being overworked when he exercised and then he didn't give them time to repair between exercises. And so they gave up. The result was that Hal had 7½ pounds less body machinery than when he started the program.

Remember: If you're in a hurry to get in shape, *exercise longer, not harder.*

We had Hal change his exercise program. He now runs four miles twice a week and at a much slower pace, so that his heart never exceeds 140 beats per minute. And he now has a stationary bicycle that he rides twice a week for about 30 minutes, again making sure that his heart rate stays at 140. When we saw Hal after another six-month interval he still weighed 150 pounds, but somehow he looked more rugged. And, of course, you know what happened. The muscles were slowly building up. He still doesn't have as much muscle as originally but with the fat content steadily decreasing and the muscle content increasing, I know he'll make it.

Figure 8. Loss of Lean Mass Due to Overexercise

Hal	Before	After (Incorrect Exercise)	After (Revised Exercise)
Total Weight	170 lbs.	150 lbs.	150 lbs.
% Fat	25%	20%	17.5%
LBM	127.5 lbs.	120 lbs.	123.7 lbs.
Fat	42.5 lbs.	30 lbs.	26.3 lbs.

10

How to Take an Exercise Pulse

I REMEMBER CAROL, a sad example of overdependence on the bathroom scales. When she first started our program, she weighed 127 pounds and was 26 percent fat. After six months of aerobic exercise, Carol had dropped to 23 percent fat. She lost two inches off her waist, two and a half inches off her hips, and one inch off her thighs. She now wore a size ten instead of a size twelve. She looked better and felt better. But when we weighed her on the scale, she had gained 6 pounds. Obviously, because of the change in measurements the 6-pound increase meant an increase in muscle mass (remember, as muscle is exercised, it becomes longer and slimmer). But all Carol could see was that she had gained weight. "This is stupid," she said and quit the program. That's what I call shallow thinking.

So, throw your bathroom scales in the dump and replace it with a new habit: taking your pulse. Your pulse is a much more accurate measurement of your health than is your weight. Most women have a resting pulse of 80 and most men average about 72. But as you become more physically fit, the resting pulse rate drops. Very athletic individuals occasionally have resting pulse rates as low as 35. Conversely, when you're ill and have a fever, the pulse rises sometimes to over 100 beats a minute.

Here are a few pointers on pulse taking. First, you'll need a watch or clock with a sweep-second hand. You can find your pulse on the thumb side of your wrist. Sometimes it's difficult to find the pulse in the wrists of women or older people, so try the side of your neck also. Lay your fingertips against the side of your neck. One of your fingers will pick up the pulse. Don't take your pulse with your thumb. It has its own pulse and you might get a double count. Once you have found the pulse, count it for exactly 6 seconds. Multiply the number of beats you counted by ten. Most people get a count of 60, 70, 80, or 90. Take your pulse again and this time be careful to note whether you were between numbers at the end of 6 seconds. You should get good enough at 6-second pulses to count half beats or even quarter beats. For example, suppose your pulse is, "One, two, three, four, five, six, and one-half." That's a pulse of 65.

This is your resting pulse. You should take your pulse several times during the day to get your *average* resting pulse. As I mentioned earlier, most women average about 80 beats a minute and men about 72 beats a minute. Here is that word "average" again. It may be average to have a resting pulse of either 72 or 80, but it would be *normal* to have a much lower resting pulse.

I have a good friend who is a superathlete. Ed missed being in the Olympics in *three* different events. One time we were camping and I decided to take Ed's pulse. At first I didn't think I had the right spot because I couldn't feel a beat. So, he tried to find it and also had trouble. Well, it turns out we didn't wait long enough. Ed had a resting pulse of 36! So I said, "Ed, what happens when you exercise?" He didn't know, but obligingly took off on a one-mile run through the woods, knocking down trees and brush that got in his way. He came lumbering back into the camp about 7 minutes later and I quickly took his pulse. It had gone all the way up to 39!

You have to picture the reserve that this guy has. Every time his heart pumps, a gallon of blood must come out. When he exercises, his heart must be saying, "Ho-hum, I guess he wants me to pump more." And out comes another gallon.

In contrast to Ed, suppose *your* resting pulse averages 100 beats per minute. Think of the implications. You have a tiny sparrow heart just fluttering away all day long. Each time it pumps, you get a thimbleful of blood. How much reserve does that frantic little heart have when you start an exercise? It would be like going down the freeway in a Volkswagen at 80 mph — and someone says "Floor it!" No wonder you get tired when you start to exercise. But if you exercise correctly and long enough, the heart muscle will get stronger and it will soon pump slower, while pumping more blood with each stroke.

You may have reacted negatively to taking the pulse for such a short count. Members of the medical profession have been so indoctrinated with the 15-second pulse that they immediately assume a 6-second pulse to be a layman's approach. I must admit that I reacted this way myself at first. But, if you want to measure your pulse during an exercise, it's usually necessary to stop the exercise momentarily. As you relax for a moment, naturally your heart starts to relax also, and your heart rate quickly slows down. If you count the pulse for the usual 15 seconds, the count will be completely false because your heart will be beating faster at the beginning of the count and slower at the end of the count. Furthermore, since the heart rate slows down more quickly as one gets in better condition, 6-second pulses become more and more important the healthier one gets.

The only exercise I can think of in which you can take your training pulse while exercising, without stopping the exercise, is stationary bicycling. When you want to check the pulse rate with any other exercise, you'll have to stop and do a *quick* 6-second count. (Remember, a 15-second pulse is not valid under these circumstances.) When you first start a new exercise you may have to stop several times to check your pulse until you know exactly how hard to do the exercise to get the correct pulse rate. After that, you should be able to do the entire 12 minutes nonstop and only check it at the end.

Fitness is **Lost** if you exercise two days or less a week.

Fitness is **Maintained** if you exercise three days a week.

Fitness is **Improved** if you exercise six days a week.

I have cautioned you many times not to drive your pulse rate above the training rate. Be sure to check your training rate often. Many people find that after several weeks of the same exercise, their hearts don't reach the training rate. Most of the time this simply means running faster, pedaling with more resistance, jumping higher, or what have you. And if this doesn't appeal to you, simply switching to a different exercise will often get your heart to its training rate.

11

Choosing an Aerobic Exercise

I MEET many people who get all fired up to begin an exercise program, only to give up after a few weeks. Inevitably, the reason turns out to be that they selected an exercise not suited for them or that they overexercised, or both. I cannot caution you too often — be sure to exercise at the appropriate heart rate! (See Chapter 8.)

I remember with horror the story of Gina. Gina was fifty-three years old with no history of exercise. But she heard me lecture and decided that running in place was going to be her exercise. When I saw her six months later she told me that she had given up after five days. She felt very guilty, but the exercise had made her so tired that she couldn't do anything for the rest of the day. When I asked her to describe what she had done, she said she had run in place for about 4 minutes and then fell on the couch exhausted. She did the same thing for five days and quit.

"What was your pulse rate?" I asked.

Well, she hadn't bothered to take it; it didn't seem important. So I had her demonstrate to me exactly what she had done. After running in place for 1 minute, I had her stop and took her pulse. It was going 170 beats a minute! This was in a woman whose recommended training heart rate is 134 beats a minute. I nearly had a heart attack worrying if *she* was going to have a heart attack! So, after a few minutes rest, I had her try again but this time she only lifted her feet about two inches off the floor. It was still too strenuous! This time her heart was going 152! Finally, I had her run in place by simply lifting her heels but keeping her toes on the floor. This exercise was enough to drive her pulse rate to 134 beats per minute. To most of us this seems ridiculous, but Gina was so unconditioned that simply wiggling her knees was an aerobic exercise.

Many people comment that they get bored doing the same exercise day after day and I would agree with them. What I am encouraging is that you do *any* aerobic exercise day after day. During the summer months you'll find me jogging on Monday, Wednesday, and Friday, swimming on Tuesday and Thursday, and taking long bicycle or canoe trips on the weekend. In the winter, it's jogging or jumping rope during the week, depending on the weather, and cross-country skiing on the weekend. Each of these exercises will result in overall, systemic cardiovascular fitness and general fat loss. Additionally, by switching exercises you avoid the problem of overdeveloping some muscles at the expense of others.

A long-distance runner's body, for instance, will adapt to the constancy of his exercise. His upper body will tend to thin out considerably. As the muscles in his arms, shoulders, and chest become fat-free they also tend to shrink a little. This does not imply that these muscles are out of condition. Muscle biopsy studies of these tissues show the extremely high enzyme counts indicative of aerobic fitness (see Chapter 26). Most runners will tell you that the sacrifice of upper body size is well worth the rewards of their sport both mentally and physically.

It's surprising how easily the aerobic exercises are assimilated into one's lifestyle. Most of them become more than an exercise. They become a sport. Daily walking or jogging conditions you for weekend mountain hiking. Daily cycling, indoors or out, primes you for weekend bike excursions in the country. There are canoe trips for the daily rower. And the camaraderie with fellow weekend runners should not be missed by the jogger. The nonaerobic exercises are pretty exclusive. It's hard to imagine a weight lifter packing a picnic lunch and going out with his girl to lift weights all day by a lovely stream. Golf? Tennis? They're great sports but not great exercise. Common sense tells us that 12 minutes of tennis or golf will hardly get us conditioned.

I'm going to discuss various aerobic exercises and you can choose one or two that are suited for you, but please don't be like

Gina. Find an exercise that gives you the correct pulse rate and save the more strenuous exercises for later.

Outdoor Aerobic Exercises

Jogging/Running

By far the most well known of the aerobic exercises, a jogging/running program will be one of the easiest to start. The only equipment you need is a good pair of running shoes. A lot will depend on how you run and where you run. In general, most of you who haven't been in a running program will be classified as joggers (there's controversy about this but as a general rule of thumb, if it takes you more than eight minutes to run a mile, you're jogging). A jogger should try to run as flat-footed as possible to avoid shin splints, jogger's heel, pulled Achilles' tendon, and strained calf muscles. Running on grass should also help if you're plagued with these problems. If you're under thirty, you can usually safely start a jogging/running program. If you're over thirty, I caution you to have a stress electrocardiogram. Those of you over fifty (and underexercised) or overweight had better look for another exercise.

Jogging and running are the aerobic exercises that result in the fastest weight loss (fat loss). I don't know why it's so, but this fact has been documented over and over again.

Walking

Walking is excellent exercise for all ages. If you're young, you may have to simulate one of the racing "walkers" to get an aerobic effect. This is a particularly good exercise for an older person since it is not as traumatic to the knees and joints as is jogging. Just be sure the walk is brisk enough to maintain your heart rate at 80 percent of maximum.

Sometimes an overweight or older person is embarrassed to jog but finds that walking doesn't drive his pulse up high enough. I solved this problem for Jane, a favorite aunt of mine. I got a small backpack and filled it with bags of sand. We experimented with different weights until we found how much she needed to carry during her walks to get the right pulse rate. Now Aunt Jane greets a neighbor while out on one of her jaunts with, "The backpack? I just returned from Europe, my dear. Simply everyone wears them there. Quite the thing, you know!"

Cycling

This is one of my favorite exercises. As a "non-weight-bearing" exercise, it's especially good for the overweight or older person. Those with back problems prefer this exercise. In fact, cyclists in general seem to be bothered less by the problems constantly plaguing runners, such as pulled muscles, twisted joints, and sore tendons. Its main drawback is locating a nonstop route so that one can maintain a steady exercise pulse. Theoretically, indoor, stationary bicycling is just as good as outdoor.

For outdoor cycling you should always invest in a good helmet. I highly recommend a ten-speed bicycle. This allows you to use the low gears when going uphill, so that you don't push your heart rate too high.

Swimming

Swimming will get your heart and lungs in excellent aerobic condition. It's also great for limbering up all the muscles in the arms and legs. I do not recommend it, however, if you're overfat. There is no reduction in fat when a person embarks on a swimming program. This has been substantiated by body fat tests done in my clinic, Stanford University's water immersion testing program, and Dr. Ken Cooper's clinic in Texas.

In contrast to the runner's body, which will shed as much weight as possible to provide more speed and agility, the swimmer's body tends to conserve its fat in order to provide warmth and buoyancy during the exercise. Every sea-living mammal has made a similar adaptation. Whales, seals, and otters have large amounts of fat covering very well trained muscles. In other words, swimming is a great aerobic exercise but you'd better add some other exercises to your program if you're overfat.

While swimming usually does not decrease body fat, I did *not* say that swimming will *add* fat. If you are 35 percent fat to start with, you will tend to stay 35 percent fat. If you are only 12 percent fat you will tend to stay 12 percent fat.

Cross-Country Skiing

The king of aerobic exercises! Unfortunately, it's seasonal. Cross-country skiing gives all the benefits of running without any of its bad effects. Instead of pounding your feet on a hard surface, you glide along smoothly. In addition, you use your arms a lot more to help move your body. A minimum of 15 minutes of cross-country skiing is recommended. (But who cross-country skis for only 15 minutes? Another plus — you tend to keep at this exercise longer.)

Roller Skating, Ice Skating

These, also, are ideal. They give the benefits of running without the trauma. But the drawback is to be able to find a rink that is not so overcrowded with people that you have to stop every few minutes. Also, be sure to check your heart rate with this exercise. It would be very easy to skate all day without getting your heart to go fast enough.

Indoor Aerobic Exercises

Everyone should select one indoor and one outdoor exercise. The indoor exercises are especially good on rainy or snowy days. Mothers with small children find it more convenient to exercise indoors. Working women like them because they generally involve less time. Many overweight people feel embarrassed doing an outdoor exercise and so like to do indoor ones until they lose some of the weight. And, if exercise bores you, you can always do an indoor exercise while watching the evening news.

Jumping Rope

This is my favorite indoor exercise. You'll need a soft surface (go to your local carpet store and get the softest remnant you can find) and a rope. I recommend that you make your own. You'll need a good ⅜-inch nylon rope and two 6-inch PVC (½-inch diameter) pipes for handles. (You can get both of these at any good hardware store.) Tie a knot on either side of the handle with just enough space so that the rope can swivel. The completed rope should come to the nipple line when you stand on it with both feet.

When you jump rope you should alternate from foot to foot at approximately 70–80 jumps per minute. Do not jump with both feet at once or try to jump faster. It's too traumatic to the feet and shins. If you need more exercise to reach your training rate, lift your feet higher rather than try to jump faster. This is one of the more strenuous exercises. Many of you may have to do several weeks of running in place before starting rope skipping.

Running in Place

This is a great indoor exercise because it can be adjusted to your physical fitness level. The really fit person will have to lift his legs high to get exercise, whereas some of you may have to be like Gina and just lift your heels. This tends to be one of the more traumatic exercises and should be done every second or third day, alternating with other exercises.

Chair Stepping

I like this better than stair climbing, which doesn't keep the heart rate steady (it slows down when you descend the stairs). This is

also a very versatile exercise in that the more fit you are, the higher
the chair should be. If you're really out of shape, try to find a
stool around five inches high. Here is the way you should do it:
Step up with the right foot, then bring the left foot up, step down

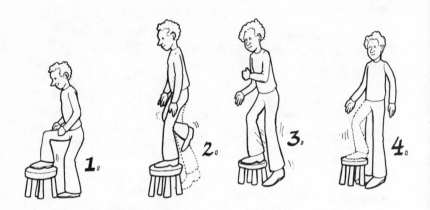

with the right foot, then bring the left foot down. With each additional step up, you should alternate feet. Be sure to keep your
back straight. This exercise is especially fun to do to music.

Stationary Bicycle

This is a tremendous exercise for the physically unfit, the older
person, or the overweight person. It is one of the few aerobic
exercises that requires some investment, however. You should
plan to buy a reasonably good one, as a cheaper model will end up
in the attic. Stay away from the motor-driven models. Also avoid
the ones that call for rowing with your arms while pedaling. I like
the ones made by the Monark and Schwinn companies. Although
it's fun to have a speedometer and an odometer, they're really not
necessary. Just adjust the tension or the speed until you reach
your training heart rate. If you're worried about bulky thigh muscles, keep the tension down and pedal faster.

Rowing Machine

Another expensive investment, but one of the best aerobic exercises. A good rowing machine will exercise almost all the major muscles of your body — your arms, back, abdomen, legs. Be sure you get one with a seat that slides so that you can push with your legs. A favorite model of mine is the Tunturi, which is made in Finland.

Treadmill

This fine piece of exercise equipment is found in many health spas. Of simple design, it is a self-powered device consisting of a slanted board on rollers with side bars for balance. A fast walk on the treadmill is comparable to a moderate jog on a level surface. Many people find that they avoid the sore knees and back associated with jogging when they switch to a treadmill.

If you belong to a spa, I highly recommend the use of the treadmill for a minimum of 12 minutes. The pace will usually be a fast walk or a very slow jog. Unfortunately, I have *never* seen a spa instructor encourage this. The usual recommendation is a fast run for 1 to 3 minutes rather than a gentle aerobic pace for 12 or more minutes. Competition seems strong in gyms, and more times than I care to remember I have seen overweight and unconditioned men running at a pace that even a seasoned runner would find difficult to maintain. Aside from the obvious danger of sudden heart attack, such headlong bursts of short but intense exercise use up the limited glucose supplies of the body, causing a temporary hypoglycemia, with its associated dizziness and nausea. Short, intense running does nothing to change the muscle enzyme chemistry necessary for the burning of fat. Only gentle exercise over long periods of time will accomplish this. So slow down and see how long you can last.

Jumping Jacks

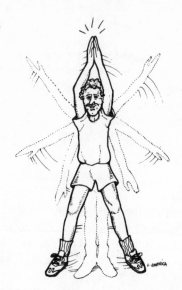

Quite strenuous, this exercise can be tempered somewhat by clapping your hands in front of you instead of overhead. This also tends to be traumatic and should only be practiced every three days with other exercises in between.

Dancing

Women especially enjoy this exercise. Do one of the popular dances of the day or create your own. Just be sure the music lasts for a minimum of 12 minutes. It's usually hard to find single records of this duration, so one woman I know tape-recorded several pieces at once and has worked out a whole routine to the music by combining running in place, chair stepping, jumping jacks, and some dance steps she made up. Square-dancing is great for older couples. See if you can get the caller to do one dance for 12 minutes during the evening.

Many dance studios now offer what they call "aerobic dance classes." The ones I've seen have been excellent. The teacher helps you determine your correct exercise pulse rate, then places you with a group of other dancers who are approximately your age and fitness. You are encouraged to check your pulse periodically while following the teacher through a series of dance steps. A friend of mine started with "The Blue Danube" and six months later was doing "The Flight of the Bumblebee"!

Mini-trampoline

The mini-trampoline is fast becoming one of the most popular forms of indoor exercise. It has been suggested that bouncing on a mini-trampoline may induce less trauma to bones, joints, and knees — particularly to people who are out of shape and not used to trauma. You can run in place on it, jump rope on it, dance to music on it.

I once spoke for an organization that placed several of these trampolines in the back of the room. When someone wanted a break, he didn't go out for a smoke. Instead, he would go to one of the mini-trampolines. I could see heads bobbing up and down as I continued the lecture. I thought this would be a distraction to the talk, but in fact it was not. When one person finished, he would be quietly replaced by another. This went on throughout the day and was one of the healthiest things I've ever seen.

For those of you who have hundreds of excuses for not exercising, think about this: I saw a man, with no legs, who regularly uses the trampoline every day by bouncing with his arms and head.

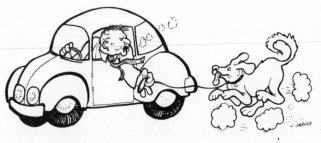

"Running your dog on a leash out the car window is great exercise . . . for the dog"

12

Heart Recovery after Exercise

ANOTHER VALUABLE CRITERION of physical fitness is heart recovery rate after exercise. There is quite a bit of disagreement as to the most meaningful way to measure this, but all physiologists agree that it's an important health indicator. After an extended exercise the heart slows down in two stages. At first there is a sharp drop, then a leveling out, or plateau, and then a slow, gradual drop to the original resting heart rate. The accompanying graph in Figure 9 is a typical example.

Figure 9. Heart Recovery after Exercise

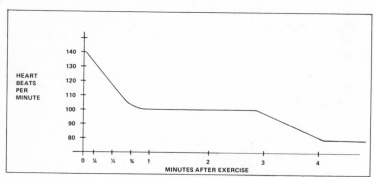

Notice that the most significant drop in heart rate occurs in the first minute after exercise. After that first minute, there is little if any change for several minutes. This resting plateau, as it is called, may last for an hour or more. Even excellent athletes may have long resting plateaus, as if the heart rate were being maintained by a postexercise emotional state rather than a physiological need for more blood. The length of time one's heart remains on the resting plateau is relatively insignificant. Therefore, the time it takes for the heart to recover all the way down to the resting heart rate is also insignificant. It's the first drop in heart rate, immediately following exercise, that is meaningful.

Some clinics measure the drop in heart rate between the end of exercise and 2 or 3 minutes after the exercise. A glance at the graph illustrates how unsophisticated this measurement is, since the critical period of recovery is in the first minute after exercise. Furthermore, it's the *slope* of the recovery curve in that first minute that matters, not simply the amount of the drop.

With practice, you can measure your own heart recovery rate almost as well as we can in our clinic. Take your pulse for 6 seconds immediately at the end of an exercise and then again for 6 seconds exactly 1 minute later. Subtract the second number from the first and divide by 10 as shown in the formula below:

Recovery Rate Formula (1 minute)

$$\frac{\text{Exercise pulse} - \text{1-minute pulse}}{10} = \text{Recovery rate}$$

If you get a high number it means your heart recovers quickly, indicating a healthy heart. There could be something wrong with your heart not shown by this test of course, but it's a good sign. Using Figure 9 as an example, an exercise pulse of 140, minus a 1-minute pulse of 100, divided by 10, gives a recovery of 4, which is good (Figure 10).

Figure 10

Recovery Rate

Less than 2	Poor
2–3	Fair
3–4	Good
4–6	Excellent
More than 6	Super!

Occasionally an individual's heart recovers so quickly that he reaches his plateau in a half minute. If you are one of these individuals, a more accurate heart recovery rate can be determined by using the following formula and then referring to Figure 10:

Recovery Rate Formula ($1/2$ minute)

$$\frac{\text{Exercise pulse} - 1/2\text{-minute pulse}}{5} = \text{Recovery rate}$$

13

Change in Muscle Shape

MOST PEOPLE expect a dramatic weight loss when they embark on an exercise program. Well, I hate to disappoint you but unless you're quite a lot overfat, there will be little if any reduction in your total weight. In fact, you may *gain* weight. Remember that muscle is much heavier than fat. As the fat is exercised away from inside the muscle, total muscle mass will increase and it's likely you'll gain 2–3 pounds. Remember, this assumes that you were not grossly overweight when you started.

What does change is your shape. Alan was a most dramatic example. Alan didn't think he was overweight but he had the middle-aged pot belly. He started an aerobics exercise program and in six months his waist went from 38 inches to 32 inches — *and he didn't lose 1 pound!* Once a woman sent me a bill for $175 as a joke. This is what it cost her to start a new wardrobe when she dropped from a size 12 to a size 8 — *while gaining 6 pounds.*

Let's look at what happens to muscle when it isn't exercised. All of us start with muscles that are long and lean with very little fat. Then as we become older and more sedentary, intramuscular fat slowly invades the muscle. The shape of the muscle itself becomes short and squat. The muscle eventually becomes so saturated with fat that it can't hold any more and then the fat begins to accumulate outside that short, squat muscle. When you diet, you lose fat from under the skin, outside the muscle. Your diet has little effect on the fat inside the muscle and nothing happens to the muscle shape. It's still short and squat. But you can exercise the intramuscular fat away and the muscle will go back to its original long, lean shape. In men, the roll around the middle disappears and women regain the waist they had in their youth.

It's the subcutaneous fat under the skin that one can see, pinch, and weigh. Obviously, loss of subcutaneous fat will result in change of body size. But usually the person's shape merely seems to be a smaller version of what it was before the loss. You go from a big pear to a little pear. It's the intramuscular fat that changes the body shape. The definition and the firmness are due to exercised muscles, not loss of subcutaneous fat. As you are exercising, keep saying to yourself, "My muscles are getting lean and slinky."

14

Should I Exercise When I Feel Ill?

EXERCISE PUTS STRESS on certain tissues and we expect those tissues to take the abuse and then recover by the time we exercise again. In fact, we hope they will repair so well that they will actually be better than they were at the beginning. In a sense, you are damaging your tissues, hoping that they will respond by getting stronger. You expect not only to repair the tissue protein that you damaged but you expect also to build some new protein. This requires protein biosynthesis, which in turn requires that your biochemistry be in good shape and that you eat some protein to provide the building blocks for the biosynthesis.

Figure 11

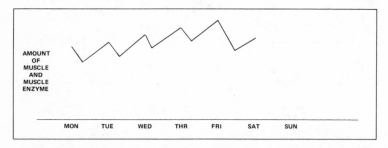

The graph in Figure 11 illustrates the way muscle and muscle enzymes can increase when a person exercises properly on a day-by-day basis. Notice that the amount of muscle and muscle enzyme decreases in the first few hours after exercise. This decrease can be measured by an increase in nitrogen in the urine over the 4 hours following the exercise. This is followed by a period of very little nitrogen in the urine as the damaged tissues absorb all the protein they can get for biosynthesis. If all conditions are perfect, the person will synthesize more muscle protein than he lost. Over several days, there should be a gradual net increase of body protein. Unfortunately, conditions are *not* always perfect. For example, the person shown in Figure 11 exercised too long and strenuously on Friday, and he was unable to resynthesize all that he lost by the time of his Saturday exercise. The result is a net loss over this 24-hour period. He might counteract this by allowing more time for the repair phase. You can see that one could have a net loss instead of a net improvement if one overexercised every day.

The body needs energy for an exercise program. If calories are limited, the protein in the diet will be converted to glucose and fat for energy, so that the protein won't be available for biosynthesis. The energy demand will always take precedence over protein biosynthesis. It's difficult to pinpoint the minimum calorie level at which protein biosynthesis can take place. I would suggest, however, that men of average size eat not less than 1500 calories while women of average size should eat not less than 1200 calories. If you are a woman currently existing on 1000 calories, I urge you not to decrease your intake as you undertake an exercise program. In fact, you may well have to increase it a bit. Superfat people in the 400-pound class must *limit* calories to lose fat, yet they must *have* calories in order to spare protein. This may account for part of the reason that these people resist weight loss so strongly. It may be that their problem is irreversible but there is no proof as yet.

In general, the older one is, the slower one's tissues repair, in the same way that cuts and bruises last longer as we get older. This means that the destruction of tissues by a hard exercise might not repair completely in 24 hours. It's quite possible to get a net loss if one exercises the same muscles too often or too hard. And with age, that possibility increases. Some people in their sixties have undertaken serious, well-intentioned exercise programs, only to have a net muscle loss because they exercised too hard or too often. Their tissue repair doesn't keep up with tissue damage.

Obviously, if you are sick, your tissue-repairing ability may be somewhat decreased. You have to decide if exercise is warranted on the basis of whether or not your "illness" will affect the same

tissues as your exercise. Take a sore throat for example. If it is
the result of shouting at a football game or too much night life in
a smoky room, it shouldn't stop you from exercise. But if that
sore throat is just part of overall aches and pains like the flu, you
had better not run. "Overall" illness, called systemic illness, will
retard tissue regeneration no matter what the exercise. By the
way, emotional stress can also decrease recuperation powers
throughout your body systems. It has been shown that the protein you eat during emotional stress is not utilized as well as usual.
During such periods, there is a distinct increase in protein waste
products in the urine.

Remember! All these factors are cumulative. If you are suffer-
ing a mild systemic illness, coupled with some emotional problems,
and a poor diet, exercise probably will do you no good. The older
you are, the more likely it is that this will take place.

Muscle Loss Will Occur If	Solution
the exercise is too intense.	• Exercise at the proper heart rate (see Chapter 8).
there is insufficient time for recovery.	• Age 30 or under — Wait 24 hours before next exercise period. • Age 30–50 — Wait 24 hours before next exercise period *and* switch exercises day by day. • Age 50 or older — Exercise every other day and switch exercises day by day.
illness or disease is present (including emotional problems).	• Lessen the intensity of exercise if you have a local injury or illness. • Don't exercise when systemically ill; the body needs the protein to repair sick tissues.
dietary protein is inadequate or imbalanced.	• Eat 60 grams of protein a day. • Be sure the diet is balanced; when carbohydrate is low, protein will be used for the making of glucose instead of tissue repair.

15

Spot Reducing

SINCE FAT CONCENTRATES in specific areas of the body, most people feel that those areas must be superexercised to get rid of the fat. Women are concerned with fat deposits on their hips and thighs and men worry about the fat around the midsection. And so they are suckered into joining health spas that guarantee to remove fat from specific areas. Or they buy all kinds of pulling, punching, kneading devices to jiggle away the fat.

There are two favorite modes of spot reducing, the passive and the active. Neither of these work! In fact, there is no known technique, short of surgery, for removing fat from any particular place on the body.

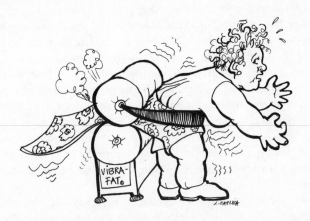

Passive spot reducers include the pulley belts and rollers often found in health spas. The theory is that if you beat it long enough, you're bound to break up the fat and disperse it. I can't help thinking that this is the way to prepare Swiss steak. You are not getting rid of the fat — you're tenderizing it. One variation of the rollers, if you can't afford to join a gym, is to simply sit on the floor and bounce up and down on your rear end. Same result — Swiss steak.

Another favorite method of passive spot reducing is a heated belt that you tie around your midsection. When it's plugged in, the heat is supposed to melt away the fat. What do you think is *really* happening? Heat and pressure drive the water out of the tissues in that area. If you remove the belt and quickly tape-measure your waist, you'll be amazed to find you've lost inches! Wait a half hour — the tide will roll in.

Another popular rip-off is the sweatsuit, a kind of cross between active and passive spot reducing. If you wear the sweatsuit while exercising, believers contend, you'll increase the burning of fat. Let me tell you, *fat boils at 360 degrees!* All sweatsuits really do is increase water loss and decrease your stamina. One of the most severe problems in long-distance running is heat prostration, in which the runner cannot get rid of body heat fast enough. When muscles get hot, the enzymes in the muscles work less efficiently. Enzymes are proteins, delicate chemicals functioning best at body temperature and body acidity. Don't try to outsmart your body chemistry by imposing artificial temperatures on it. Wear enough clothes to be comfortable. The best method is to wear layers of clothing and shed the outer garments as you warm up.

It also follows that it would be foolish to try to lose weight in saunas or steam baths. These are simply other methods of manipulating body temperature. At best, it's unwise if done in excess (you may be destroying those delicate muscle enzymes needed to burn up fat) and can be downright dangerous if your body is trying to fight off an infection or virus (your temperature will already be elevated). And, of course, any weight loss will be water loss, not fat loss.

Now what about active spot reducing? In general, this involves using the muscle that is directly beneath the fat deposit. I'll have to admit I was conned into this myself. I was starting to get a little roll around my midsection so I did what anyone would do.

Sit-ups. I did 300 sit-ups a day. I did sit-ups first thing in the morning. I did sit-ups on my coffee break. I'd stick my feet under the tracks and do sit-ups while waiting for the trolley. I'd even hang by my legs from an exercise bar and do sit-ups. Within three months, my stomach muscles were like cast iron . . . but with three inches of marshmallow on top of the muscles.

Women frequently complain about fatty deposits on their upper thighs. So they do leg raises and donkey kicks or they buy pulleys that loop around the foot, over a door, and are attached to a weight. They work that poor muscle to death.

Now in both of these cases, sit-ups and leg exercises, what you are essentially doing is a weight-lifting type of exercise. And when a muscle is exercised by weight lifting, it enlarges (hypertrophies). The end result is a *larger* muscle with that same fat deposit sitting on top of it. The subcutaneous fat lying on top of a muscle doesn't "belong" to that particular muscle. It belongs to the entire body. And it's only going to get used up if the caloric demand is so great that the fat is needed for fuel. When only one muscle or a relatively small set of muscles is exercised, the caloric demand is small. But when large sets of muscles are exercised, the fat will be drawn from all parts of the body to meet the energy requirements. And the largest sets of muscles in the body are in the legs and buttocks — the very muscles used in any aerobic exercise.

The point of all this is — it is impossible to reduce subcutaneous fat from a selected spot on the body. It simply cannot be done! One can reduce the intramuscular fat by selective exercising of one area but this will not affect the fat deposited under the skin lying over those muscles. Subcutaneous fat must be thought of as "belonging to" the whole body. Food in the icebox doesn't "belong" to the cook just because the cook is near the icebox all the time. Fat under the skin, like food in the icebox, is stored for "general use." One person, no matter how gluttonous, will take longer to clean out the icebox than a whole bunch of hungry, but normal, eaters. One muscle, no matter how much it is exercised, will take longer to use up the fat on top of it than will a whole bunch of exercised muscles. Get your largest muscles all going at once if you want subcutaneous fat to decrease.

In women subcutaneous fat is deposited first at the back of the thigh, then on the outside of the thigh, then the hips, then the midriff, and finally in the upper body, particularly under the arms. In most cases, these subcutaneous deposits are removed in reverse order. If you are a woman with fat in those places, and you start a daily bicycle exercise program, the fat will decrease in reverse order from the way it was deposited. Even though bicycling is basically a leg exercise, you will lose fat from your arms first and your legs last.

No matter how many times I tell people to lose fat by systemic (aerobic) exercise, someone inevitably asks how to lose fat from some specific place on the body. Women with fat arms seem to be convinced that arm wiggling, or rubbing, or pounding, or push-ups is necessary to get the fat off their arms. Believe me, if you bicycle or jog, that fat will drain away a lot faster.

That special puckering in women's legs, often called cellulite, is just lots of fat under a slightly different skin texture. It may be driving you crazy but I warn you not to be suckered into exercises or manipulations of that particular area. Remember, the only people who worry about unsightly fat in one area are people who constantly do things to change that one area. People who get involved in whole body athletics, and particularly aerobic exercises, trim down all over without getting "hyper" about the fat in any one place. And, of course, good athletes are never concerned about specific fat deposits.

16

Weight Lifting

As STATED in the previous chapter, exercising isolated muscles in the body will do little to decrease the fat around those muscles. Fat deposits are only decreased with systemic (whole body) exercise. However, weight-lifting exercises are good for local muscle changes. A person can increase size or strength of specific muscles. For instance, skiiers often do squats with barbells on their shoulders to increase the strength of the thigh muscles. The pectoral muscles across the front of the chest can be enlarged through proper weight lifting. These muscles support the breasts, giving women an opportunity for dramatic change in their figures. Many runners do upper body weight lifting to counteract the natural thinning that goes with their sport. Weight lifting is also the best approach for the occasional person who is trying to gain weight.

Weight lifting doesn't have to require barbells and dumbbells. Bags of sand, large cans of food, or heavy books work quite well for the beginner. Even push-ups and sit-ups are good weight-lifting exercises. If your arms or abdomen are just too fat, do an endurance exercise to reduce them. Then add push-ups or sit-ups to strengthen the muscles.

The next time you are in a gym or spa, ask yourself as you start each exercise whether the exercise is going to have systemic or local effects. Is it basically an aerobic, low intensity, long-term exercise, or is it basically weight lifting, lasting only minutes, requiring pretty heavy effort? The short-term weight-lifting exercise burns almost no fat from any part of the body. A few calories are used, of course, but they will be glucose calories rather than fat calories, and there is recent biochemical evidence that intense glucose burning actually stimulates synthesis of fats in the muscle.

Take sit-ups as an example. Let's say that you see someone (either male or female) with a very attractive body, including a nice flat abdomen, and the person says, "I do lots of sit-ups." Don't be fooled into thinking that all you have to do is sit-ups to duplicate that figure. The person is doing several other things of a systemic, fat-removing, nature that he may or may not be aware of. The sit-ups make the abdominal muscles strong, which helps to control posture and even to prevent lower back problems. I highly recommend them. But they don't remove fat.

Now you can see the folly in attempting to reduce flabby thighs by swinging heavy weights with your legs. Such effort is too short in duration to burn significant calories and may well increase the size of the muscle, making the leg even bigger.

Aerobic endurance exercise should be a must in any weight-lifting program. Use weight lifting for strength and bulk. Use endurance exercise for weight control and fitness.

17

Don't Confuse Work with Exercise

ONE OF MY GOOD FRIENDS, Tim, who is a long-distance runner, recently bought a farm in Oregon. I saw Tim a few months after he moved and asked how he was feeling. "Out of shape," Tim replied, "I've been working so hard that I'm not getting any exercise!" Sounds strange, doesn't it? Tim was up every day at dawn, feeding the animals, milking the cows, plowing the land, piling bales of hay. By the end of the day he was exhausted — yet he didn't feel exercised!

Remember, very few calories are used during any exercise. Be it weight lifting, aerobics, or something else that somebody dreams up, very few calories are used *during the exercise*. But! Exercise changes us. It increases the metabolic rate, increases the amount of muscle, raises the level of calorie-consuming enzymes inside the muscle, and increases the burning of fats. Sustained exercise at 80 percent maximum heart rate is very efficient at bringing about these changes. Most jobs involve short bursts, which are inefficient at bringing about these changes. Yes, physical work is a form of exercise, but, like weight lifting, it is not effective weight control.

A frequent complaint I get from women is, "Exercise! I exercise all day long! I chase the kids, and mow the lawn, and do the dishes, and the cooking, and the housekeeping. Why I never stop exercising!" When I tell them that they're not getting any exercise at all, they're ready to slug me.

I realize this might sound confusing but look at it this way. Suppose the muscle in your arm was capable of lifting 60 pounds. Now all day long you are working that muscle. The housewife will lift 20 pounds of laundry, 15 pounds of groceries, push that muscle to do ironing, gardening, maybe even to spank her kids. But at no time during the day has she put a *sustained* demand on her body. To the muscle, it's just busywork. She's tired at the end of the day, but the muscle has only been worked to about 50 percent of its capacity. Hence, 50 percent of the muscle can turn to fat. The work you do may cause the heart to beat faster, but you rarely sustain the work long enough to get any benefits. Work, in fact, should be put in the weight-lifting or sprinting category. It is non-aerobic. It is usually of too high or too low an intensity or of too short duration to produce the desired metabolic changes.

Additionally, work usually demands one set of muscles. Aerobic exercises put a demand on all the muscles of your body, including the heart muscle. You may not think your arms are getting any exercise when you are running but, metabolically, they are getting conditioned. Aerobic exercises will get you in condition for work, but work won't get you in condition for exercise.

One of the fattest men I've known was a physician in Sacramento, California. When he was ten, his father died, and from that age on he had to support himself. He had done all kinds of strenuous labor from carpentry to hod carrying. Even after he had worked his way through medical school and could afford to sit back and relax, he still kept right on working in every spare moment. When I tested him in the water tank, he came out 55 percent fat! How do you tell a man like that that all that work doesn't amount to a proper exercise?

18

Insensible Exercise

FIT PEOPLE often get involved in exercise without *sensing* that they're doing exercise at all. In other words, their fitness allows them to do physical things without being aware of it. We call such unconscious muscular activity "insensible exercise."

It's popular in books on dieting to knock exercise. "Exercise doesn't burn enough calories to be of any significance," the diet books often say. And to prove it, they use this example: "Jogging burns 9 calories per minute. The average person jogs 20 minutes for a net loss of 180 calories, which approximates the number of calories in a glass of milk."

These numbers are correct. That's right, very few calories are used during exercise. But exercise changes us so that we burn more calories throughout the day, even if we aren't deliberately exercising. For example, exercise warms the body and the warmth lasts long after the exercise is over. When the body is warm, there is a slight increase in the metabolic rate, indicating a slight increase in calorie burning.

Metabolic rate can be measured with a portable oxygen tank similar to the tanks and hoses that skin divers use. One exercises or simply carries out daily chores while breathing oxygen. Since oxygen is used in the body for the burning of calories, the amount of oxygen used per minute tells us how many calories a person is using.

Let's contrast two accountants, the same age, weight, and height — everything identical except that one jogs for 20 minutes before work and the other doesn't. For the first working hours each day our jogger will be warmer and burn more calories than his colleague, even if they do identical work. This is often called an "exercise high."

By the way, drug abuse is much less common in physically active youngsters, just as alcohol abuse is much less common in physically fit adults. An "exercise high" is all the "high" that fit people need. And an exercise high makes you healthier, whereas a drug high does the opposite. Think about that the next time you come home from work and think you deserve a little liquid high.

It can also be shown that physically fit people have slightly elevated metabolism. Even when they are at rest fit people burn more calories than fat people do. Exercise is cumulative. Instead of counting the number of calories you burn each time you exercise, concentrate on the extra calories you will burn two years from now, even when you are asleep.

Take two housewives, the same age, height, weight — everything identical except that one is fat and one is fit. The fit woman's "dish-washing metabolic rate" will be higher than that of her fat counterpart. When both women go out grocery shopping the fit one will be using slightly more calories than the fat one. And so it goes with every other activity. The fit woman's "ironing metabolic rate," "cooking metabolic rate," and "window-washing metabolic rate" will always be a fraction higher than the fat woman's.

Time and motion studies have been done to show these differences in activity level in another way. Movies were taken of high-school girls at recess playing volleyball, tennis, and basketball. Later, in a laboratory, the films were slowed down and each individual still was labeled as to whether the girl was active or inactive. During all sports, the fat girls had a significantly higher percentage of inactive time than did the fit girls.

Have you ever watched two fat people playing tennis? They have the longest arms! They have become so efficient that they hardly move at all. Fat people have adapted to a low "activity metabolic rate" so that they don't really do as much during any given exercise. They unconsciously find ways to get the same job done with less movement. So when our fat housewife is washing dishes, she is using fewer calories because she has become efficient, unconsciously, in finding ways to eliminate unnecessary movement. It's only in the more active sports that this efficiency of motion becomes clear and in the very active athletics, it becomes a detriment — they can't compete.

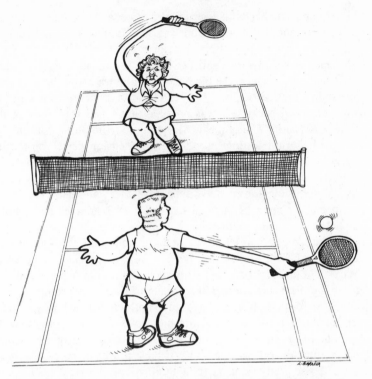

**"Have you ever watched two fat people playing tennis?
They have the longest arms!"**

In other words, fit people are inclined towards insensible exercise. They're the ones who shift in their seats during the sermon in church. They're the ones who get up and go to the refrigerator instead of asking the spouse to bring them something. They're the ones who join their kids in a game of Frisbee when the family is on a picnic instead of sitting on a blanket with the Sunday newspaper.

Not only do fat people unconsciously move less, but I've met some who are downright sneaky in finding ways to avoid exercise. I worked in a San Francisco weight clinic in which all the clients were at least 60 pounds overweight. I remember the day I had Marjorie use the stationary bicycle. I got her all adjusted on the bicycle and left her with instructions to pedal five miles. I turned to counsel another woman and was surprised when, what seemed like only a few minutes later, Marjorie appeared at my side. "I'm all done," she said with a satisfied smile. It seemed to me that Marjorie had only been on the bike about 3 minutes. And, besides that, she didn't look very sweaty. Well, I didn't want to accuse her of not exercising because it was possible that I had lost track of the time, so I said, "That's great, Marjorie, show me how you did it." What Marjorie had done was loosen the tension device on the bicycle to zero resistance. She then straddled the seat, gave the pedals one good kick and stuck her feet out as the pedals whizzed by. When they slowed down, she gave them another kick to get them going again. "I pedaled five miles in 3 minutes at 90 miles an hour!" she said proudly.

In the same weight clinic we used to do an initial test for physical fitness by having the person walk a mile as quickly as possible. We would give the person a stopwatch and a map depicting an exact one-mile route around the streets of San Francisco. We had to find a route that didn't have any shortcuts because people used to cut through alleys, crawl through holes in fences, anything to get out of going the whole distance. It took some of the people 45 minutes to walk a mile. They'd have to rest at every telephone pole. I got pretty good at judging how long it would take a particular person to walk the course and when Dorothy came into the clinic, I figured she would be gone so long that I would have time to go out for lunch. Well, it's a good thing I didn't take that lunch break because Dorothy was back in 12 minutes! She had taken a taxi! Honest! She got down to the first corner, decided this was not her style, and hailed a cab back to the clinic.

The point then is that exercise for a few minutes a day, by altering our insensible exercise for the rest of the day, has far-reaching effects. Claiming that jogging for 20 minutes is ineffective because it burns only 180 calories is grossly misleading.

19

Sing Praises to Protein

PEOPLE KNOW that fat is especially concentrated in calories, so if they are trying to lose weight, they avoid fat. If we add to this the common misconception that carbohydrate is fattening, they also begin to avoid carbohydrates. That leaves protein. In America, everybody eulogizes protein. It started with the reports about protein starvation in India and Africa. Then our coaches and athletes got wind of the idea that muscle is made from protein — and the rush was on. Now proteins are associated with health, life, all kinds of good things. Even hair spray is sold by its protein content. Hot dogs are criticized for their low protein content. Weight lifters pour protein powder in their egg nogs and on their ham sandwiches.

So, naturally, the most popular weight loss diets push high protein, and low carbohydrate and fat. But how do you get a high protein diet? By eating lots of meat, right? Well, in case you haven't noticed, meats, particularly in America, are very high in fat. In fact, it's the fat content that makes our meats taste so good. The more expensive the steak, the more intramuscular fat in it. That means that a high-protein diet is really a high-protein *and* fat diet. In fact, the most popular low-carbohydrate diets contain so much meat, and therefore so much fat, that they are higher in calories per mouthful than a high-carbohydrate diet.

People do lose weight on high-meat/low-carbohydrate diets, however. One reason is that fat in food delays digestion quite a bit, so you feel satisfied with less food. Another reason for their seeming effectiveness is that high-protein consumption tends to cause loss of body water. If you lose ten pounds on a high-protein diet, two or three of those pounds may be water of dehydration.

Later, your body reabsorbs the water and you regain that portion of your weight loss, making the diet much less effective than it seemed.

But this isn't the major criticism of high-protein–fat/low-carbohydrate diets. The big danger is that they are conducive to muscle loss and to degeneration of muscle tone and efficiency.

Since fat, carbohydrate, and protein are the only sources of calories in the diet, the various weight loss diets consist of an endless list of manipulations of these three foods. What few people realize is the wondrous way the liver manipulates these foodstuffs for you. Once digested and in the bloodstream, they are carried to the liver, which readily converts one to another (Figure 12). Your body needs

Figure 12. Possible Interconversions of Foodstuffs in Liver

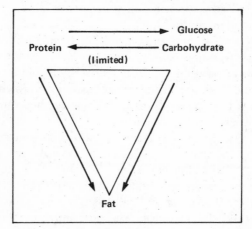

all three, of course, and the liver is so sensitive to those needs that it starts interconverting very quickly if you eat a particularly unbalanced meal. It is as if your liver were saying, "Go ahead, dummy, eat that ridiculously unbalanced meal; I'll straighten it out." You may have some smart new idea that your body needs less of this and more of that, but believe me, your liver is a lot smarter than you are.

The interconversions that are possible in the liver are shown in the accompanying triangle (Figure 12). Notice that although many interconversions are possible, there are no arrows leading away from fat. Fat is never converted into protein or carbohydrate. I drew the triangle when I was in a pessimistic mood, with fat at the bottom to indicate that excesses of anything in the diet can lead in a downhill direction — to fat. And who wants fat in the bottom! The only thing your body can do with fat is burn it up in the muscles (Figure 13).

Figure 13. Pathways for the Burning of Fat, Glucose, and Protein

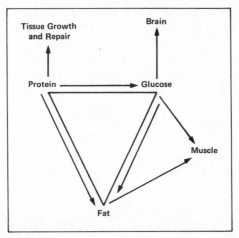

Notice, also, that protein can be converted into glucose. Most of the time, when people think of glucose, they think of muscle because muscle burns glucose for energy. But muscle can exist without glucose. The essential thing about glucose is its use by the brain. The brain must have its glucose! Ask anybody who suffers from hypoglycemia how they feel when their blood sugar is low. They get woozy, dizzy, and sometimes have blurred vision. When you are not exercising, your brain uses two-thirds of the glucose in your blood. Just think what that means — an organ weighing only 1–2 pounds burning up 66 percent of your circulating glucose while your 30–70 pounds of muscle scrapes up the rest. In other words, when you are not exercising, 1 pound of brain burns sixty-six times as much glucose as 1 pound of muscle. The brain is quite a glucose hog. Furthermore, the brain won't function without its glucose, but the muscles will! If you exercise too much, your muscles use too much glucose and your brain experiences the symptoms of sugar shortage that I just mentioned. This is one of our built-in safety mechanisms. I'm sure that when the good Lord made us, He knew that we would be foolish creatures, the only creatures who think that exercise to the point of exhaustion is play. So, if we go too far, we faint from lack of brain food. It's hard to exercise when one is unconscious, so the liver gets a chance to build up the glucose supply by converting protein to glucose.

The point of all this is to emphasize that the conversion of protein to glucose is a powerful body function, one which operates if you should endanger blood glucose supply in any way. For many years it was assumed that the glucose that is stored in the liver, called glycogen, was the principal source of blood sugar between meals. But it has been shown recently that this glycogen is hoarded by the liver. Instead of giving up its glycogen for blood sugar, the liver converts protein to glucose.

If you subsist on a bare starvation diet, either voluntarily to lose weight or involuntarily, as in a prison camp, you will convert valuable body protein to blood sugar for your brain. You will lose muscle, the very tissue you need most to burn up the food you eat. If the diet is low not only in calories, but also extra low in carbohydrate, you will lose body protein even faster. Typical high-protein/low-carbohydrate diets are usually as low in total calories as a prison camp diet and they are devastating to body muscle if practiced for any length of time.

It seems odd that a diet that emphasizes protein would cause a loss of body protein, but it does because the total calorie intake is so low. For up to 2 hours after a meal, your body can use the protein in that meal to make glucose if the carbohydrate in the meal was low (a rather expensive way to get your blood sugar), but after that there isn't any more dietary protein in spite of the fact that you may have had a high-protein meal. Two and a half hours after a meal, all of the protein in that meal has been used in some manner and is no longer available for the production of glucose. Now how is the brain going to stay alive until you feed it again? The answer is that the body will feed on itself. It will break down its own muscle tissue (protein) and make it into glucose. This process will occur whether you eat a balanced diet or an unbalanced high-protein/low-carbohydrate diet. But the hooker is this. The protein that you eat should be used to repair the tissues that have been broken down during the time you weren't eating. Instead, in the high-protein/low-carbohydrate diet, the protein is needed immediately for the production of glucose and the muscle tissue does not get replaced. (In a well-balanced diet, the carbohydrate in the meal will be used for glucose production, leaving the protein available for the muscle repair.) The net result of a high-protein/low-carbohydrate diet is that the muscles break down and are not repaired, with a consequent loss in Lean Body Mass. As I said earlier, it's possible to lose as much as 1 pound of muscle for every pound of fat on one of these diets.

Most experts agree that approximately 60 grams or 2 ounces of protein a day is enough to meet the needs of the body *and* supply the additional protein needed just in case the person is also lactating, pregnant, has the flu, a broken leg, and is lifting weights. A high-protein diet that contains excess calories such as used by weight lifters who are trying to *gain* weight will not cause a loss of muscle.

What happens when you eat too much protein? You can't repair any more tissue than that which needs repairing and you aren't going to grow a new foot, so obviously the body doesn't need the amino acids. And when amino acids aren't needed, they're sent to the liver where they're deaminated and then converted into FAT. Not only that, the process of deamination (when your body has to do a lot of it) can be stressful. During deamination the nitrogen that is released from the amino acids is quickly converted into ammonia. Ammonia is very toxic to the body so it in turn is changed into urea. Urea is also toxic, to a lesser extent, and to eliminate it from the body, it must be diluted into urine. In a normal, balanced diet in which protein constitutes about 12–13 percent of the total caloric intake, your body can very easily rid itself of the urea. But what happens when you suddenly increase the protein intake? You've got to get rid of the urea and you're going to need enormous amounts of water to dilute it. You may drink a lot more water but it won't be enough. Inevitably, your body will have to take water from its own tissues to dilute the urea. You've suddenly put a very stressful burden on your kidneys, which are working overtime to get rid of the urea. Oh yes!, you're losing weight like crazy, but most of it is water loss. Your body may lose up to 12 pounds in water alone on a high-protein/low-carbohydrate diet, regardless of how much water you drink.

How can one be sure to get enough protein in the diet while also getting a good balance of carbohydrate and vitamins? A reasonable rule of thumb would be to eat two servings daily of 3 ounces of a meat product (preferably low-fat meats such as chicken and fish) or, better yet, a meat substitute (split peas, dried beans, lentils). In addition, have two servings (1 cup each) of nonfat or low-fat milk or a milk substitute such as yogurt, low-fat cottage cheese, or cheese (one slice is a serving). Balance these high protein foods with carbohydrate by eating four servings of fruits/vegetables each day and four servings of high roughage breads and cereals, which are grain products (discussed in Chapter 23). To determine a serving size of fruits/vegetables or of a grain product, picture the food broken up into bite-size pieces. If it would almost fill a cup (¾ cup) then it's a serving.

While it's important to balance your diet with adequate amounts of protein and carbohydrates, you will not have to worry about getting enough fat. It is almost impossible *not* to get fat in the foods you eat. Even if you decide to eliminate all animal products that are high in fat, you would still get fat in nuts and other seeds such as the wheat germ.

20

Do Muscles Burn Fat or Glucose?

THE MAIN FUNCTION of fat is its use by the muscle for energy. Almost all diets prey on the misconception that it is hard to burn fat. The fact is that when you are not exercising, 70 percent of the energy need of muscle is met by fat and only 30 percent by glucose. It's not hard to burn fat, we burn it all the time.

Think about it this way; suppose your weight has been stable over the last six months. There has been no gain of weight and no loss of weight. Where has all the fat gone that you have eaten each day? You put butter on bread, oil on salad, and eat fat in all meats. Each day you may have eaten 500 calories of fat, some hidden and some obvious. That's equivalent to 60 grams or 2 ounces. If you haven't gained weight, then where did all that fat go? Well, it's consumed by muscle metabolism.

Fat has one dominant function, to provide energy. It can be burned, metabolized, oxidized, call it what you will. There is no better source of energy for your body than fat and we burn off quite a lot all day long even if we are not exercising. Competitive athletes, particularly runners and cyclists, have the idea that their muscles run on glucose because blood glucose levels drop very low during competition and contribute to fatigue. They correct this by eating some sugary food or drink, which further convinces them that it's glucose that makes their muscles go. The truth is, the muscles burn a combination of fat and glucose and if it weren't for the fat supply, our athlete friends would run out of glucose in just half the time. The only reason they notice the glucose loss is because they run out of it. It isn't likely that they will run out of fat. And here lies both the beauty and the drawback to fat. It's such an efficient, beautifully stored energy source that we never run out of it even though we burn it all the time.

Frank Shorter, America's great Olympic marathon runner, reportedly has 2 percent body fat. He weighs 135 pounds, which means his body contains about 3 pounds of fat. You would think this might be a drawback for him, since he will want all the calories he can get during a marathon run. But! One pound of fat amounts to 3500 calories, so his three pounds of fat amount to 10,500 calories. In a 2½-hour marathon run, his muscles consume about 800 calories per hour, or 2000 calories, and only 50 percent of that is fat. In other words, he burns up less than ⅓ of a pound of fat during the run.

The runners who have the most energy left at the end of a long run are not the ones who stored the most glucose. They are the ones who are best adapted to using fat as energy during the run, thus saving their limited glucose. If women dominate the long-distance running world some day, it will not be because they have more fat in their bodies but because they are better able to burn fat during the stress of exercise.

The difference between fat and glucose might best be explained by an analogy. Let's imagine building a fire in your fireplace. If you put in a big log and light a match, what happens? Nothing! The match just goes out. So you put some twigs of kindling wood under the log and light the kindling wood. Well, glucose is like kindling; it is easy to burn. Fat, on the other hand, is like a log; it is hard to get started and won't burn well unless some kindling is added once in a while. But it burns for a long time, giving off lots of heat.

Fat, like logs, contains lots of calories. To keep fat burning properly, you need a little glucose to act as kindling. If your muscle cells receive only fat, they can burn it, but they burn it incompletely, giving off half-burned waste products called ketones, much the way a log starts to smoke if you don't put some kindling under it once in a while. These ketones end up in the urine just the way smoke comes out of a chimney. One popular diet suggests that lots of ketones in the urine shows lots of fat is being burned. What does it mean if lots of smoke is coming out of a chimney? Does it indicate a big fire inside? Of course not! It only indicates a poor fire that smokes a lot. Ketones in the urine indicate *poor* combustion of fat, rather than *lots* of combustion of fat.

Glucose, like kindling wood, is good for quick energy, but, like kindling wood, it doesn't last, so its total calorie value is limited. We use glucose exclusively for energy during a sprint. There just isn't time to get those fat logs burning.

Short-distance runners are glucose burners. Long-distance runners are fat burners.

The enzymes in muscle that burn glucose are quite different from those that burn up fats. For some reason, the fat-burning enzymes seem to be particularly fragile. As one gets out of shape (and fat), the ability to utilize fats for energy decreases rapidly, leaving the glucose-burning enzymes to carry on. One of the characteristics of being out of shape, then, is that one uses blood glucose while resisting the use of fat. Hence, the more fat you have, the less fat you burn.

Referring to the triangle discussed in Chapter 19, and also to Figure 14, let's see what happens when a fat person exercises

Figure 14

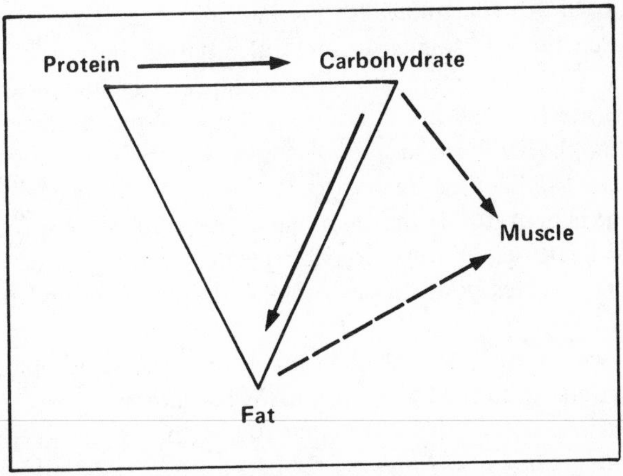

heavily. Keep in mind that for the fat person, walking to the icebox may be heavy exercise. During the exercise, the fat person's muscle burns mostly glucose, since fat-burning enzymes are lacking. This brings down the blood glucose, a temporary hypoglycemia. Exercise stimulates hunger in a fat person, while athletes experience a decrease in hunger after exercise. The fat person's hunger may well be due to the low blood sugar, although this has not been proven. In any case, he eats, and usually some carbohydrate food is included. The carbohydrate becomes blood glucose, which rises abnormally high, due to his insulin insensitivity (Chapter 27). The high blood sugar, having trouble entering the muscle, enters fat cells instead, where it is converted into triglyceride.

In other words, the fat person who exercises heavily resists burning the fat he is trying to get rid of and then makes more fat right after the exercise. He could react to this by refusing to eat any carbohydrate after exercise but this would not alleviate the blood sugar problem. The liver would then convert protein into glucose, so he would lose more muscle. And, horror of horrors, he may even lose more of the enzyme proteins — the very proteins he needs to encourage the burning of fat.

The proper way for the fat person to counteract this vicious cycle is as follows: First, exercise very mildly over long periods, because mild exercise allows for the burning of a higher percentage of fat. Second, eat some carbohydrate, but of the complex type (Chapter 23) that enters the bloodstream slowly. Third, eat this carbohydrate in small quantities six or more times a day.

Let's emphasize once more that "mild" exercise, being a relative term, is best defined as exercising at less than 80 percent of your maximum heart rate. It makes no sense to try to burn off fat with bursts of exercise, because you are burning pure glucose. Long, slow exercise gives your muscles time to burn off fat and minimal glucose.

In seasoned athletes, particularly those who do aerobic sports such as running and cycling, this circle is quite reversed. In fact, they have a circle of their own that is just the opposite, and it is not vicious. They resist making fat and at the same time burn fat readily. During exercise, the athlete is able to rely on stored fat for calories, thereby saving precious glucose. As mentioned, the exercise does not induce hunger, but if the athlete does eat some carbohydrate food, blood glucose will take a more moderate rise because much of it quickly enters the muscle cells to restore muscle glucose (glycogen). Furthermore, his blood glucose levels remain more uniform and this eliminates the need for any conversion of valuable protein to glucose. Thus, the athlete's dietary protein can be used exclusively for its intended purpose, repair and synthesis of body tissue.

Since fat people use up their limited glucose supplies more quickly than fit people, their blood glucose levels tend to be low more often. This will obviously affect the incidence of hypoglycemia, and even diabetes. Both of these diseases are much more common in fat people and it is probable that they are related to poor muscle enzymes rather than weight. Every physician knows that borderline diabetes in adults diminishes if the patient loses weight, but these patients should be encouraged to lose fat rather than weight and also to increase the fitness of their muscles.

At this time, mild diabetes and hypoglycemia are treated with diet, the main mechanism of which is to reduce and control carbohydrate intake. This does alleviate the symptoms but it's not in any way a cure. If you stop eating carbohydrate because your body can't handle carbohydrate, it's similar to treating a broken leg by saying "don't walk on it." I don't claim for a minute that exercise will cure all blood sugar problems, but the evidence is good that training your muscles to burn fats readily can decrease rapid plunges in blood glucose.

The sad thing about the grossly obese people who often claim they would do anything, absolutely anything, to lose weight is that they refuse to do the one thing that will do them some good. They refuse real exercise, possibly because they associate exercise with sweat and exhaustion. But you see now that the fatter and more out of shape one is, the slower the exercise should be. They must avoid intense exercise like the plague because it will only burn off sugar. For the very fat, seemingly mild exercise such as walking quickly may in fact be excessive. Their fat-burning enzymes are so poor that even the slightest effort shuts off fat consumption. If I were grossly fat, I would give up whatever was necessary — job, housework, whatever — and I would walk three to four hours per day. I would never give myself a chance to rest, but I would be supercareful not to exceed 80 percent of my maximum heart rate.

Superfat people may take three-quarters of an hour to walk a mile while good athletes can cover the same mile in 4 minutes.

Obviously, there is a vast difference in their muscle chemistry. For such fat people, and the eminent scientists who counsel them, to continue to blame their eating habits for their obesity is clearly ridiculous. There are 500-pound people who are getting fatter every day on 1000 calories while undergoing psychological counseling and behavior modification to convince them to eat less. And so they eat less and less, starve themselves more and more, and get fatter and fatter. It is impossible under such starvation circumstances to synthesize the very enzymes they need to reverse their condition. They get weaker and weaker, progressively losing the desire and the ability to do the one thing that would do them the most good. There is even a club of fat people now whose leaders have pledged to retaliate against society's discrimination of the obese by not exercising at all. Good luck to them!

21

Is There Anything Good about Fat Storage?

YOU BET there is! For those creatures that have to move about the earth for food and sustenance, fat is the greatest thing ever invented. You see, all living things, even plants, have to store a certain amount of food for the days when they can't find or make food. So they store calories either as carbohydrate or as fat. But carbohydrate is a very bulky, heavy form of calories, too cumbersome for mobile creatures. Carbohydrate is stored only by plants, which don't need to move, while all animals store calories in the form of fat.

Most people know that fat contains about twice as many calories per pound as carbohydrate; but there is another, more important reason to choose fat as a stored energy if you must move (Figure 15). When carbohydrate is stored in the body, inside cells, it is

Figure 15

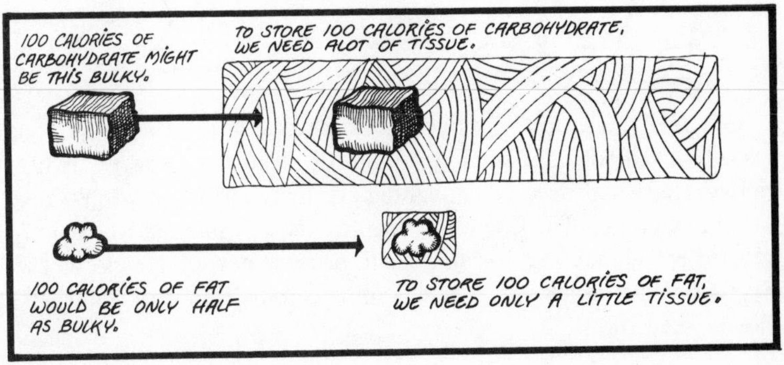

100 CALORIES OF CARBOHYDRATE MIGHT BE THIS BULKY.

TO STORE 100 CALORIES OF CARBOHYDRATE, WE NEED ALOT OF TISSUE.

100 CALORIES OF FAT WOULD BE ONLY HALF AS BULKY.

TO STORE 100 CALORIES OF FAT, WE NEED ONLY A LITTLE TISSUE.

stored in the form known as glycogen. Glycogen can occupy only about 15 percent of the space inside a cell. The rest of the cell must be left to other functions, most of which require a watery medium. Fat cells, on the other hand, can contain 85 percent fat, leaving only 15 percent cellular space for the water-based life functions of the cell. This means that fat is not only twice as caloric as carbohydrate but much more of it can be packed into a small space.

The result is that body fat, being 85 percent pure fat, and highly caloric, contains about 3500 calories per pound. Contrast this with the liver, which stores glycogen carbohydrate at only 250 calories per pound. I once calculated that if I were not going to eat for three weeks but I wanted to start out with enough stored calories to last for the whole period, I could either take 9 pounds of fat around my middle or the same number of calories as glycogen in a 126-pound liver (and presumably a wheelbarrow).

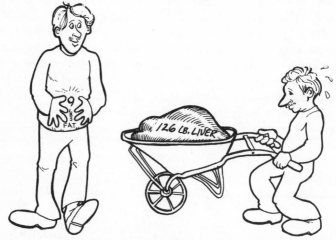

Obviously, a mobile creature is far better off with this marvelous invention called fat. Plants store almost all of their energy as carbohydrate, which is no disadvantage to them since they don't have to go anywhere. The one exception to this is in plant seeds that are carried by wind, water, or animals to become new plants elsewhere. Seeds contain much fat: hence, safflower oil, peanut oil, and sunflower seed oil.

There is also an exception in the animal world. Clams and other shellfish that lie in wait for their food may seem fat but, in fact, they are not. They store energy as carbohydrate since the neat compactness of fat is no advantage to them.

Plants were the first living things. After a while, the plants started crawling around on land and we called them animals. This means that carbohydrate was first in evolution, fat appearing only when animals appeared. Hence, fat has a higher evolutionary status. If you are fat, you may derive some consolation by telling your friends that you are unusually high on the evolutionary scale.

Since fat is so neat a bundle of calories, higher animals have evolved many ways of making it. The body can make fat out of protein. The body can make fat out of carbohydrate. And the body can make fat out of fat; that is, fats in the diet from plant seeds or meats can be processed into human fats. In other words, almost everything you eat, if it can be digested at all, can be converted to fat. That's where the problem comes from; fat is such wonderful stuff that humans have evolved many efficient pathways for making it. Fat people are particularly efficient at doing this.

You must realize that the ability to store food, in any form, is a great advantage to any creature. It is like having money in the bank, because it increases your options in life. You should consider stored fat as a safety mechanism. In earlier times, man was, like other animals, occasionally forced to endure short famines. In those times, he could, like the camel, live off his hump. Man, being a high evolutionary species, has evolved many biochemical routes or pathways for the synthesis of fat and has evolved complex biochemical routes to circumvent the use of that fat and hence to save it.

It has been postulated that one of the reasons fatness is a problem today is that we have inherited the ability to deposit fat very easily. The theory is that our cavemen ancestors often had to go days between meals. The ones that survived were probably the ones whose bodies were somehow able to adapt to the harsh conditions. And one way of adapting was to carry a little extra fat that the body could live on. Naturally, these primitive men didn't look fat. They were much too active. But they passed on that ability to store extra fat. The body you have today is still watching out for that possible famine and carefully conserving a few calories out of every meal to be tucked away as fat.

The point of this chapter is to emphasize that your body visualizes fat as a physiological safety mechanism. Physiological stresses are countered with an increased depositing of fat and a decreased utilization of stored fat. While research has not shown that *every* stress induces this response, many are known. It seems prudent to avoid bizarre weight loss schemes because the body reacts by increasing fat storage even though you may be losing weight.

There is, for example, good evidence that the popular high-protein/low-carbohydrate diets actually increase the percentage of your diet that is made into fat while you are losing weight. After several months on such diets, even if you have lost 30 pounds, your body has changed, so that you have a fat person's chemistry. Your tendency to get fat is greater than when you started!

The one thing that most fat people are eager to do is lose weight rapidly, but rapid weight loss by any method also induces the change to a fat person's chemistry.

Fasting is another stress that has been shown to make you fatter while you think you are getting thinner (Chapter 22).

Remember, fat is actually very good stuff. Your body will react to radical behavior by attempting to make more fat, even if you are losing weight.

22

Fasting

THE BODY IS STRESSED when it is deprived of food and will try to lay down extra fat for the emergency. In other words, *fasting will encourage your body to become fatter.* A study on rats illustrates this phenomenon. Fifty rats were separated into two groups. Both groups were given exactly the same daily quantity of food. Group A rats ("Nibblers") could eat the food all day long but Group B rats were allowed only a one-half hour feeding to consume all the food ("One Big Mealers"). It took the One Big Mealers a little while to get used to it, but once they realized that no more chow was coming for twenty-three and one-half hours, they gobbled up all of the allotment in the half hour. The amount of food was low enough that both groups lost about the same amount of weight.

At the end of six weeks, the rats were allowed to return to a normal amount of food and the One Big Mealers were allowed to be Nibblers again. Both groups gained weight. The One Big Mealers gained slightly more weight than the Nibblers. The researchers analyzed those enzymes in the rats that are responsible for the depositing of fat. Enzymes in the One Big Mealers had increased nearly tenfold during the low-calorie diet period. Even though the rats were losing weight because total caloric intake was low, it was as if their bodies were saying, "The minute more food comes along, I'm ready to lay down extra fat just in case this stress happens to me again!" In the first part of the experiment, when both groups were losing weight, the Nibblers had no increase in fat-depositing enzymes.

In other words, if you *have* to diet, don't make the mistake of fasting or eating just one meal a day (essentially a 23-hour fast). Spread those calories out over the day in five to six small meals.

Otherwise, you're setting your body up for a heavy fat gain the minute you go off the diet.

This increase in fat-depositing enzymes doesn't last forever. They eventually go back to normal if you stop dieting. But, in the rats, it took eighteen weeks to go back to normal — three times the amount of time it took to get them out of balance.

Now if you can visualize that fat was originally meant to be a marvelous advantage to mobile creatures and that it represents a magnificent safety device against famine, you can appreciate that the body will attempt to make more of it under most stress circumstances. Temporary fasting is a stress! Even eating only one meal per day is translated by the body as a 23-hour fast, causing a higher percentage of the food you eat to be made into fat. Hence, less food is available for energy and tissue repair. Likewise, most diets that are high in protein and low in carbohydrate are translated as an emergency situation, bringing an increase in the depositing of fat.

23

People Are Eating Too
Much Carbohydrate! Right?

In AMERICA, in the early 1900s, 10–12 percent of the average American's calories came from protein, 60 percent from carbohydrate, and 30 percent from fat.

Figure 16. Percentage of Daily Calories

	1900	1970	Recommendation
Protein	10–12%	12–14%	12%
Fat	30%	44%	23%
Carbohydrate	60%	44%	65%

While eating patterns have changed quite a bit since then, you might be surprised to learn that protein consumption has changed only slightly. Americans still get about 12–15 percent of their calories from protein. But! The amounts of both carbohydrate and fat have changed. Are we eating more carbohydrate — or less? Most people are quick to say that Americans are eating much more carbohydrate than before and that is bad.

In fact, carbohydrate consumption has *decreased* drastically from 60 percent of the day's calories to about 45 percent. Sugar, which is only one form of carbohydrate, has *increased* drastically, thanks to soda drinks, cookies, cakes, and the hidden sugar that is added to many foods. While sugar consumption goes up, overall carbohydrate consumption is going down. People seem to be afraid of bread and cereal and vegetables. These contain the complex forms of carbohydrate, called polysaccharides. You are thinking of starch, right? There is starch in bread, potatoes, and cereal. But starch is only the beginning of the complex carbohydrates. There is cellulose, hemicellulose, and lignin, which are only partly digested. These are the materials of roughage that we hear so much about. We are urged to eat more roughage, but nobody ever mentions that *roughage is carbohydrate.* It is odd that while carbohydrate has almost become a dirty word, roughage has become a magic word. Yet they are the same thing. There is a great deal of difference between one carbohydrate and another, even though all carbohydrates have certain chemistry in common. For example, all carbohydrates, after intestinal digestion, become the simple carbohydrate called glucose. It's just that some carbohydrates break down in the intestine very quickly, some very slowly, and some (like cellulose) not at all. This means that the complex carbohydrates will become blood glucose very slowly while the simple sugars such as maltose, lactose in milk, and table sugar will become blood glucose almost immediately. Complex carbohydrates may even decrease the availability of the sugars in a food.

The people who encourage us to eat roughage are right. We should eat more of that form of carbohydrate. We should decrease the amount of simple carbohydrate because simple carbohydrates are, in a sense, predigested and cause our blood glucose levels to fluctuate too quickly. My urging is that we increase our carbohydrate consumption but only by eating more of the complex variety.

Let's look at the variety of carbohydrates found in just one food such as corn in the form of corn on the cob. As you can see from Figure 17, one kernel of corn contains the full range of carbohydrate complexities. When tables of nutrient content were first derived, corn was determined to be only 2 percent indigestible because hemicellulose and lignin were not yet recognized. In those days the corn was put into a glass, ground up, and "digested" with acids and alkalies found in the laboratory. After the digestion, 2 percent was left. Recently, however, independent laboratories in England have done a more realistic digestion of the corn using actual digestive enzymes from the human digestive tract. With these methods, 12 percent was left as indigestible, and further research exposed a whole new set of carbohydrates called lignins and

Figure 17. Complexity of Carbohydrate in Corn

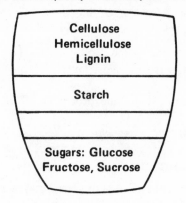

hemicellulose. In other words, corn is much less digestible than the nutrition tables have indicated.

Most people have noted from personal experience that corn doesn't digest very well.

Corn is a type of cereal grain, as are rye, wheat, rice, barley, and oats. All of them have similar characteristics, with the roughage carbohydrate forming the outside layers. The outside layers of wheat kernels can be cracked off in tiny flakes called bran. Bran is nothing more than the roughage carbohydrate from wheat. You would think there was something magical about it the way it's pushed by nutrition authorities. But bran is only one form of roughage. The roughage from other cereals is just as good. Furthermore, if you are increasing roughage in your diet by sprinkling bran on other foods, you are not getting the rest of the nutrition in the wheat kernel that is found underneath the bran.

The studies from Africa showing the advantages of a high rough-age diet do *not* extol the virtues of pure roughage; it's roughage *foods* they are talking about. Africans, protected from colon cancer, diverticulitis, and appendicitis, do *not* sprinkle bran on their Cheerios. They eat the bran still attached to the rest of the wheat kernel; that is, they eat whole wheat. Some primitive, high-rough-age cultures eat wheat, some eat corn, some eat rice; but all of them eat the grain in a relatively whole, unrefined condition close to the way it's grown. In this way they get the full gamut of carbohydrates shown in Figure 17, plus the vitamins and minerals associated with each of the carbohydrate layers. By eating the whole grain, they get several benefits:

1. The caloric value of the food is decreased by the roughage.
2. Roughage is hard to chew, thus decreasing the tendency to overeat.
3. The roughage gives some protective effect to the digestive tract.
4. They eat their vitamins *with* their food as nature intended.
5. The simple sugars give taste but are delayed in their entrance to the bloodstream.

I don't condemn adding bran to your diet but, even though bran itself is a natural substance, it's another artificial way of supplementing a poor diet. It would be better to increase roughage carbohydrate through whole grain breads and cereals, adding as few fats and sweeteners as possible. Too many people are continuing to eat highly refined sugary breads and cereals while sprinkling bran over them as if it were a panacea.

From the foregoing it is clear that the American mania against carbohydrate is ill founded; that Americans are eating less and less total carbohydrate while increasing the sugary sweets. We should make every effort to reverse these two trends.

24

How Much Fat
Are Americans Eating?

HAVING SET THE RECORD straight that Americans have been decreasing the total carbohydrate consumption, we can now question fat consumption. It surprises most people to learn that we have increased our fat consumption (see Figure 16 in Chapter 23). In fact, fat has increased from 30 percent daily calories in 1900 to approximately 45 percent today. One of the main reasons for this is the increased availability of high-grade meats. Even if all the fat is carefully trimmed away, the remaining marbled fat, much of which is invisible, would still constitute 30 percent to 50 percent of a piece of steak. It's surprising, but it's the high-income people, the ones who can afford the filet mignons and the prime ribs, who eat the most fat. Wild animal meat, or at least range-fed cattle meat, is lower in fat and would be better for us.

The proliferation of margarines has also contributed to the increase in fat in our diets. People have been lulled into thinking that only saturated fats such as butter are harmful and, as a result, have increased their consumption of unsaturated fats. Five or six years ago scientists thought that the unsaturated fats were not conducive to arterial plaque formation. Now they're not so sure. Evidence now points to the fact that unsaturated fats, although causing a decrease in blood cholesterol, cause an increase in the amount of cholesterol in the arterial plaques, artery walls, and other body tissues. Unsaturated fats probably play just as great a role in heart attack as do saturated fats. It would be far better to decrease *all* fat intake.

In Chapter 23, I emphasized the need to increase complex carbohydrates. Well, if we increase the percentage of carbohydrate calories that we eat, clearly the percentage of something else must go down. We should decrease dietary fat as much as possible. It is almost impossible to eat too little fat. I could almost urge you to try to eat no fat at all because I know that you would inevitably get enough fat hidden inside your foods. For practical advice, however, I urge that you eat a minimum of meat, particularly red meats, which contain so much fat, both obvious and invisible. In addition, decrease the use of fat in cooking and put less butter and margarine on foods.

The oils, margarines, and fats that we use in food preparation are similar to refined sugar in food value. For example, safflower seeds in their natural form may have a reasonable food value, but when we squeeze out their oil to make safflower margarine, we leave most of the nutrition behind and are left with pure fat (or oil). Similarly, we can get corn oil from corn, peanut oil from peanuts, and for that matter, butter from milk. These fats and oils are almost pure grease and we don't need them. Unfortunately, sugars and fats make food tasty. It will be hard for all of us, but we are going to have to get used to eating less of both of them.

25

The Big Picture

UNFORTUNATELY, many of the questions that arise from a book like this can only be answered by a discussion of the chemical reactions that take place in a muscle cell. There are whole books written on the subject with titles like *Intermediary Metabolism* or *Physiological Chemistry*. Believe me, they don't make for pleasant Sunday afternoon reading. Nonetheless, I am going to try to give you a quick overview of the chemical reactions involved in a muscle cell as it attempts to extract energy from all that food we eat. Chemists will criticize me for oversimplification. But we can criticize them for making this important information so sticky that it isn't any fun. If you get bogged down reading it, I don't blame you. Just pass on to the next chapters and come back to this one after your next aerobic exercise when your brain cells are better oxygenated.

Glucose from carbohydrates, fatty acids from fats, and amino acids from proteins are burned inside muscle cells to get energy. But what does "burn" really mean in this context?

"Burning," in a muscle cell, doesn't fit the image most of us have of burning. Let's pretend you have a small wooden building in your backyard that is no longer useful and you decide to disassemble it in order to make use of its lumber for other projects. You would have to do the job carefully, step by step, in order to avoid ruining each piece of lumber. It would be much simpler to touch a match to it and burn it down, except that you would have no lumber for your other projects. Cellular burning is more like taking a building apart, a careful procedure requiring special tools called enzymes for each step.

It's important that you realize the significance of the enzymes involved. Literally hundreds of these fancy tools are needed in each cell and each one is quite different from the others. Each enzyme is made of protein. They are large, complex molecules that cannot pass through the wall of a cell. Because an enzyme molecule is so large, it would be folly to think that enzymes added to the diet or injected into the bloodstream will end up in muscle cells. The only way enzymes increase in a muscle cell is when the DNA *makes* more enzymes inside the cell. This is called enzyme biosynthesis and takes place only if you eat adequately, if your cells aren't sick, and if you exercise to stimulate the DNA to go to work.

Enzymes are delicate proteins. While all tissue proteins in the body are continuously broken down and repaired by DNA, the enzyme proteins break down the quickest. If you don't exercise, the DNA doesn't repair them as fast as they break down and your ability to burn calories decreases.

The burning (or disassembling) of glucose in a muscle cell takes place in two stages. During the first stage the glucose is broken down until it becomes pyruvic acid. In the second stage the pyruvic acid is completely disassembled into water and carbon dioxide (Figure 18). Enzymes used during the first stage need very little

Figure 18. Energy Production inside a Muscle

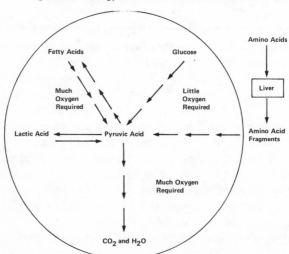

oxygen to do their work. Hence, this stage is referred to as the anaerobic phase ("an-" meaning without). The enzymes that function during the second stage need lots of oxygen, so this is called the aerobic phase.

We have defined aerobic exercise as exercise in which the heart rate does not exceed 80 percent of maximum. At this pulse rate the heart and lungs are able to supply‾enough oxygen to the muscles so that glucose can be disassembled through both stages and can be completely burned. If the exercise causes the pulse rate to exceed 80 percent of maximum, then the heart and lungs cannot keep up with the oxygen demand in the muscle. When this happens the glucose will only be broken down to pyruvic acid. There will not be enough oxygen to continue through the second stage. Exercise that exceeds 80 percent of maximum is called anaerobic exercise. Since pyruvic acid cannot be burned during anaerobic exercise, it accumulates in the muscle and is converted into lactic acid. Excess lactic acid in the muscle is painful. The pain is often so intense that you can't continue the exercise. As you "catch your breath," oxygen flows into the deprived muscle One-fifth of the lactic acid turns back into pyruvic acid, to be burned aerobically. It has been postulated that the other four-fifths is converted into fatty acids.

We find that there is a completely different set of enzymes used for the burning of fats. Fatty acids, either from our fat deposits or from a recent meal, are carried by the blood to muscle cells. Inside the cell, the enzymes are lined up ready to take the fatty acid apart and get the energy out of it. Each enzyme does its work in an orderly sequence that biochemists call a chemical pathway. If you look at Figure 18 you will see that the first half of fat burning, called the Beta oxidation pathway, is unique to fats. The second half of fat burning uses the exact same enzymes as the second half of glucose burning.

Unlike glucose burning, in which the enzymes require little oxygen in the first stage, all the enzymes used in fat breakdown need a lot of oxygen. Anaerobic exercise, therefore, effectively shuts off all fat burning and forces the muscle to use glucose exclusively. The 80 percent maximum heart rate that I have been pushing not only allows you to burn fat while exercising, but also stimulates DNA synthesis of more of these enzymes. As the enzymes proliferate, you are able to grab oxygen from the blood better and better and use fats at higher and higher exercise intensities. That is, you will be able to run faster, yet still run aerobically and burn increasing amounts of fat!

Notice in Figure 18 that amino acids are also burned in muscle by the oxidative enzymes. This means that proteins can be burned along with fats and carbohydrates. This often occurs in people on very low-calorie diets. The body can't get enough energy from fats or glucose and therefore burns valuable protein instead of using it for tissue repair.

Heavy weight lifting is on the extreme end of *an*aerobic exercise, whereas walking is perhaps on the extreme end of aerobic exercise. The trouble comes when we try to distinguish between exercises that are somewhat in the middle. For example, if I go out for a jog or a slow run, which type of exercise am I doing? The answer lies in whether I am running out of breath or not; whether I can continue on and on or have to stop. Theoretically we could say to you, walk, jog, or run as fast as you can without getting out of breath, without feeling exhausted when you quit. But this technique hasn't worked well in practice because people who hate exercise quit when they have run out of breath mentally, while some people won't slow down for anything because they won't even admit to themselves that they are out of breath.

This latter group of diehards or "jocks" are almost always men with an athletic past. They are the ones who overstress themselves to their own detriment, as explained in Chapter 9, and who break up marriages by exhorting their wives to "Run faster, honey! Can't you keep up?!"

The best way to know for sure that you are exercising aerobically is to exercise at 80 percent of your maximum heart rate as discussed in Chapter 8.

I'm afraid that I have to admit to belonging to the jock group myself and I will tell you an embarrassing tale to make a point. In graduate school at M.I.T., I played a lot of hard squash and I was quite good at it. Squash, like racquetball and handball, is really a series of short *an*aerobic bursts. An hour of that game will exhaust almost anyone. So I thought I was in great shape. Once in a while I played with a dentist friend named Lou who preferred to run but who enjoyed our occasional games of squash. I could usually beat him but was always surprised at how well he played and how long he could last despite playing so rarely. One day Lou talked me into going for a long, slow run with him. After about half a mile, I had to stop and vomit. I didn't seem to have any guts for it. Well, now I know what was going on. Lou's aerobic running got him in shape for my sport but my *an*aerobic sport wasn't getting me in shape for his.

One of my main reasons for writing this chapter is to point out the importance of muscle enzymes, particularly the fat-burning enzymes. If you haven't got enzymes, you are going to get fat. Enzymes will increase only if you stimulate the DNA by exercise and if you eat enough that there will be amino acids available for biosynthesis.

26

Muscle, Its Enzymes, and Mitochondria

I HAVE SUGGESTED repeatedly that exercise alters muscle metabolism in such a way that fit people can eat more without making more fat. To understand this, let's think about muscle for a moment. Muscle is unique in its ability to produce sudden bursts of energy. All cells require energy, but cells other than muscle undergo relatively small changes in their energy requirement. For example, brain cells use only two times as many calories during intense thinking as during sleep. Muscle cells, on the other hand, going from a resting condition to a sudden burst of energy, may increase their energy demand by fiftyfold in a split second. Obviously, the nutrients that have filtered into the cells from the blood will supply the source of energy, just as with other types of cells. Only in muscle cells, however, can one find enzymes competent to metabolize the nutrients so quickly. In blunt terms, muscle has special enzymes enabling it to burn up tremendous amounts of calories in short periods. It's the only tissue with enzymes that are specialized for sudden increases in calorie burning. This alone would be enough to convince me to keep my muscle in tone, just on the possibility that there might be more enzymes in there waiting to consume a passing calorie.

Remember, also, that muscle constitutes a large portion of the body, between 30 and 50 percent. Now let's put together three important facts about muscle. First, muscle uses many calories because movement is more calorie-demanding than any other body function. Second, muscle uses many calories just because a large percentage of the body is composed of muscle. Combine the first two factors and you can see that of all the calories burned in the body, 90 percent are burned by muscle, even if you are sedentary. When we add the third fact, that specialized enzymes, existing only in muscle, can increase calorie burning by fiftyfold during exercise, the 90 percent figure becomes more believable. Clearly, if you want to get rid of calories, you should look to the quantity and quality of your muscle.

Suppose that through radical dieting you lose a small percentage of your muscle. And suppose, through the same radical dieting, you also lose some of the enzymes in the remaining muscle. Such fractional losses add up to a significant decrease in your ability to burn calories, so you get fat more and more easily. Clearly, dieting will not increase muscle and it will not increase enzymes inside the muscle.

Most of these particular enzymes are located in a special place inside muscle cells. They are found in the mitochondrion, a potato-shaped object, many of which can be found scattered throughout each individual cell. That's where the metabolizing enzymes are located and, if you want to burn up calories, that's where the action is. It has been shown repeatedly that steady aerobic exercise actually causes an increase in the number and size of mitochondria in each muscle cell. Further biochemical studies have confirmed that, with exercise, there is an increase in metabolizing enzymes inside those mitochondria.

Enzymes are proteins, very complex fragile proteins that are put together out of dietary amino acids inside each cell. These proteins, even more than others, are continuously broken down and rebuilt. This process is easily thrown out of balance. People who are getting in shape with regular exercise are increasing these enzymes. In people who are getting more out of shape day by day, the enzymes aren't needed, so they are slowly discarded.

We have all seen pictures of skeletonlike people coming out of prison camps and the haggard look of someone who has lost weight too quickly. Most of us have seen how dramatically an arm wizens if put in a cast for six months. These are familiar examples of tissue protein loss that are easy to visualize. The loss of protein in the form of enzymes is much less obvious but of the utmost importance. A loss of several pounds of muscle is bad enough but the loss of one ounce of muscle enzyme is drastic.

27

Insulin Insensitivity

I HAVE STATED that fatness is a vicious cycle; that is, as one gets fat, the body changes to favor getting still fatter. The condition known as insulin insensitivity partially explains this phenomenon. It was observed some time ago that in fat people, blood glucose levels and insulin levels are unusually high after eating carbohydrate. In all people, eating carbohydrate causes a rise in blood sugar, followed by a rise in blood insulin, which the pancreas produces to handle the sugar. In fat people both of these responses are abnormally high. The reason is that the fat person's tissues are insensitive to his own insulin.

All body cells are impervious to glucose until insulin comes along and stimulates them to open certain pores, which then allows the entrance of glucose. If it weren't for insulin, all the cells of all your tissues would starve for glucose no matter how much glucose was in the bloodstream. As one gets fat, it goes without saying that one's muscles get out of shape. In so doing they lose their ability to respond to insulin. This means that glucose can only enter the muscle cells very slowly. Since muscle accounts for 30–50 percent of the body, blood glucose levels remain elevated longer after a meal. This means extra glucose is circulating around in the bloodstream looking for some other cells to enter. And what kind of cell does the fat person have lots of? Right! The sugar dumps into the fat cells. With the muscle cells rejecting the glucose, the fat tissue becomes a glucose sink.

The question is, "So what?" We are concerned about *fat* accumulating in fat tissues, not *glucose* accumulating in the fat tissue. The trouble is, inside fat cells glucose is converted to glycerol and glycerol attaches to three fat molecules. Glycerol plus three fatty acids is called triglyceride, which is the neutral, stable kind of fat that body fat is composed of. Glucose becomes the skeleton for fat formation.

To review: As one gets fat, muscle changes. One of the changes is that muscle becomes insensitive to insulin, hence rejecting glucose, which then piles up in the fat cells to foster the growth of more fat. The paradox then is that the person with the least need for more fat makes it the fastest.

28

Contradictory Advice

THE READER will undoubtedly encounter information that seems to contradict what you have read here. Be sure to find out if the advice or research that is being offered pertains to fat people or fit people. For example, my cautions regarding exercise, especially not to overexercise, are intended for that 99 percent of the population not involved in competitive athletics. You will hear coaches pushing interval training, also called wind sprints. This technique can be applied to many sports but, illustrated with running, it involves running as hard as you can for perhaps 100 yards, followed by jogging until you get your breath back. Without ever stopping, you alternate jog and sprint. This technique is well proven to be effective training for competitive athletes. But it doesn't apply to the other 99 percent of us. It doesn't even apply to the author at 13 percent fat, running six miles a day, four days a week. I'm not into competition; I just want to be healthy.

The point here is that many techniques will be thrown at you over the years that may well be effective for the trained athlete but not for the other 99 percent of the population. Even fasting, which I totally discredited in Chapter 22, may have some benefit to marathon runners. Their bodies handle such stress quite differently. Sugar consumption is still another case in point. Unquestionably, we all eat too much of it, it devastates the teeth, and it promotes a host of other problems. On the other hand, for seasoned athletes in the midst of competition, a mouthful of sugar is a great help.

Here is another confusing issue. Research studies done by top scientists at Harvard have shown that a ten-week exercise program has no effect on obesity. If you read the study, however, you find that they started with people averaging 450 pounds and 80 percent body fat. Ten weeks of exercise, the researchers claimed, did not diminish the tendency of the subject to get fat. Well, of course not! The subjects may have dropped to 75 percent fat, but they were still very fat people with fat people's chemistry. They were still insulin insensitive and still unable to metabolize fats. Exercise for such obese people only reduces subcutaneous fat and has little effect on musculature. Furthermore, when fat people exercise, it increases their hunger.

Even advice on warming up before exercise and cooling down after is confused by the well-intentioned but mistaken coaches. If you are going into a competitive event, it is bound to be at maximum stress, which is *an*aerobic. Under *an*aerobic stress, blood flow to the digestive organs is greatly restricted and digestion can be impeded. So, if you undertake a *hard* run right after breakfast, you may well get sick to your stomach. Similarly, kids who go swimming right after a meal may be more likely to get cramps, since most kids swim with *an*aerobic bursts. But I am urging gentle aerobic exercise! Radical changes in blood flow, digestion, and adrenalin secretion are not typical during aerobic exercise. A sensible meal followed by aerobics is okay in most individuals. Warming up and cooling down (Chapter 7) are good but much less critical than claimed by those who are used to the problems of competition.

Let's assume that 1 percent of the population is extremely athletic and into competition. Let's also assume that about 4 percent of the population is grossly obese, more than 100 pounds overweight. That leaves 95 percent of the people in the United States in the middle who will not go wrong following the advice in this book. Unfortunately, most of the advice on exercise comes from the competitive 1 percent, so it doesn't apply to the majority of us. Most of the research and advice on overweight comes from work with extremely fat people who abhor exercise, and that doesn't apply to you and me either.

29

Why Not Now?

I WON'T TELL YOU that getting used to daily exercise is a bed of roses. There are times when the best of us would rather quit, put up our feet, and dream of a diet or a pill that will make us healthy. But health doesn't come in a bottle or a diet.

Even the best diet combined with the most potent vitamins will never tune up your muscles the way good exercise will. It seems a shame to put expensive fuel in a poor machine. If your car isn't running well, do you drive all around town looking for a better and better gasoline, or do you have your car tuned up? Remember, it's your muscles that burn the vast majority of the calories you eat. It's largely your muscle chemistry that determines whether that good diet or those vitamins get properly used or just wasted.

It would be nice if everyone had the opportunity to get weighed under water occasionally to determine just how fat one is. Lacking this information, it's impossible for you to know whether you are overfat or not. Occasionally we see people in our clinic who look overfat but who are just big-boned and big-muscled without much fat at all.

The point is, it is impossible for me to tell you in a book what weight to shoot for; but it is equally impossible for you or your doctor or a table to tell you what weight to shoot for. If you have been reading this book thoughtfully, you should be convinced by now that the cause of excess fat is poor muscle tone. You should shift your thinking from weight to things associated with muscle. You should think about your level of physical fitness and measure changes in that.

Don't ask how much you should weigh. Stop shooting for an ideal weight! Shoot for health; for being physically fit. When you exercise, don't think about how many calories you are burning; think about your enzymes. When I do my morning run, I mutter under my breath, "Grow you enzymes, grow!" If you can, check your blood pressure once in a while to see if that comes down as you get healthier. By all means check your resting pulse. The easiest thing of all to check is your measurements. The waist of both men and women decreases as the abdominal mucles flatten out. Hip and thigh measurements in women decrease quickly with exercise.

These simple measurements may seem unsophisticated but they are far better measures of health than your weight. If you want more encouragement, ask your doctor if there are other things that he might check from time to time. For instance, if you tend to have a trace of sugar in your urine, it will decrease with good exercise. Hypoglycemia decreases with exercise, as does high blood triglyceride. Don't get anxious — these improvements take time, at least a year, sometimes four or five years in older people.

Having tuned-up muscles doesn't mean that you have to become an athlete. It means more energy, more drive, better utilization of food, and less conversion of food to fat.

So, start exercising! Like the rest of us, you will falter from time to time, but persist, and gradually your whole physical and mental well-being will improve. Be sure to "pulse-monitor" your efforts so that you won't overdo, so that you can dodge much of the muscle pain that used to be a regular part of unguided exercise. Reversing twenty years of fatty muscle degeneration may take months, even years in some cases, but hang in there; lots of us are with you. I mean, *really* with you.

Join those of us who are proud to be getting the most out of the bodies we were given. Start now!

The Aerobics Logbook

Twelve-Month Program

A Realistic Approach to Exercise

The Aerobics Logbook is for everybody — young, old, male, female. It is carefully designed so that you can achieve maximum physical fitness with a minimum of stress. The emphasis is TIME, not distance.

Too often, people who want to improve their physical fitness quickly make the mistake of overexercising by exercising too hard. Most exercise programs stress distance and time relationships — how far can you run, jog, cycle, row, or whatever in a certain time? You are led to believe that improvement comes only when you shorten the time it takes to do a certain distance. Inevitably, competitiveness causes you to overexercise.

Studies have shown that, for the greatest improvement, the heart should only be stressed at 70–80 percent of its maximum potential. Stressing the heart beyond this can result in decreased physical fitness and may actually be harmful. Improved physical fitness comes with lengthening the exercise, not by trying to do more work in the same amount of time. Remember, if you want to get in shape fast, EXERCISE LONGER, NOT HARDER.

You will notice that in this logbook there are no spaces to keep track of distances covered. The only way you get "points" is for the time spent exercising, at the proper heart rate. If you're out of shape, it may take you 20 minutes to cover a certain distance.

A friend may be able to complete the same distance in 10 minutes. If you both have been exercising at the proper heart rate, you'll earn more "points" because you exercised longer. Your friend will have to do twice the distance to earn the same points. Of course, as you get more fit, you'll be able to cover greater distances in the same time. BUT! You'll earn more points only when you spend *more time* exercising. Therefore, you should only be concerned with two things when you exercise:

1. How long did you exercise?
2. What was your pulse rate during the exercise?

When you exercise for a certain amount of time only and forget about the distance, you will have two advantages. First, you don't need to find a measured course or track. All you need is a wristwatch. You can go anywhere. Second, you aren't tempted to exercise too hard. There is no final destination you are trying to reach. If you decide to run or cycle faster it won't make any difference. The time won't go any faster. If you are shooting for a certain distance, you'll try to go faster to get it completed. But you can't hurry up time. No matter how slowly you go, time passes at the same rate.

The Aerobic Exercises

Aerobic exercises are unquestionably the *most efficient* exercises to improve physical fitness. You will show greater improvement with aerobics, *per time spent,* than with any other exercise. Therefore, unless you have lots and lots of time to spend exercising, save the tennis games, handball, skiing, weight lifting, or golf for fun and do the aerobics for exercise.

An aerobic exercise is one which:

1. is steady and nonstop
2. lasts a minimum of 12 minutes
3. maintains your heart at 70–80 percent of maximum for the entire time you are exercising
4. should be done a minimum of four days a week.

AEROBIC	NOT AEROBIC
Walking	Downhill Skiing
Running	Tennis
Jogging	Handball
Bicycling	Racquetball
Rowing	Weight Lifting
Cross-Country Skiing	Calisthenics
Dancing	Golf
Jumping Rope	Sprinting
Roller Skating, Ice Skating	

How to Determine Your Training Heart Rate

You should learn how to determine your: Resting Heart Rate, Maximum Heart Rate, and Training Heart Rate.

1. Resting Heart Rate: Take your pulse for 6 seconds and multiply by 10. Most people will get a 60, 70, 80, or 90. Take your pulse again and this time notice whether you are between counts on the sixth second. If you are, then your pulse will be 65, 75, 85, or 95. You should take your pulse several times during the day to determine your average.

2. Maximum Heart Rate:

220 minus Your Age = Maximum Heart Rate

This is the fastest your heart can beat for your age.
DO NOT EXERCISE AT THIS RATE!!!

3. Training Heart Rate:

[(Maximum Heart Rate minus Resting Heart Rate) × 65%]
+ Resting Heart Rate = Training Heart Rate

Example: A forty-year-old has a resting heart rate of 70. To calculate his training heart rate: $(180 - 70) \times 65\% + 70 = 141.5$. When this person exercises, he should maintain a heart rate of 141–142 beats per minute.

When you exercise, check your pulse immediately at the end of the exercise. (Count it for 6 seconds and multiply by 10.) If it's going 10 or more beats slower than your calculated training heart rate, you're not exercising hard enough. If it's going 10 or more beats faster than your training heart rate, SLOW DOWN. Remember, you're working *with* time, not racing against it.

Aerobic Exercise Categories

I	II	III
Required Minimum Time 12 Minutes	Required Minimum Time 15 Minutes	Required Minimum Time 20 Minutes
Jumping Rope Running in Place Jumping Jacks Chair Stepping	Jogging Running Cross-Country Skiing Rowing Dancing	Walking Outdoor Bicycling Stationary Bicycling Ice Skating, Roller Skating Swimming

You can see from the categories that, to acquire the same result, some exercises require more time than others. Twelve minutes of jumping rope is equal to 15 minutes of jogging or 20 minutes of cycling. This is because Category I exercises are the most strenuous and Category III exercises are the least strenuous. Obviously, if you decide to do only Category III exercises you would be spending more time than a person who only does Category I exercises. In order to compare accurately one exercise to another, we modify the time spent in any one category by a "fudge factor" for that category.

Example: Suppose in one month, you spent a total of 90 minutes doing exercises in Category I, 150 minutes doing exercises in Category II, and 200 minutes doing exercises in Category III. This would be a total of 440 minutes but the ADJUSTED TIME would be only 412½ minutes:

$$
\begin{array}{lll}
\text{Totals:} & \text{Category I} & 90 \times 5/4 = 112.50 \\
& \text{Category II} & 150 \times 1 \ \ = 150 \\
& \text{Category III} & 200 \times 3/4 = \underline{150} \\
& & 412.50 \ \textbf{Total Adjusted Time}
\end{array}
$$

You can see that 90 minutes of Category I exercises will earn you 112.5 "time points," whereas 200 minutes of Category III exercises will be reduced to 150 "time points."

Fitness is **Lost** if you exercise two days or less a week.

Fitness is **Maintained** if you exercise three days a week.

Fitness is **Improved** if you exercise six days a week.

Before you start . . .
1. Check your resting pulse. (It will decrease as you become more fit).
2. Calculate your training heart rate. _____ = Training Heart Rate.
3. Check your measurements:
   Waist _____ Hips _____
   Right Thigh _____ Right Upper Arm _____
4. Weight _____

Suggestion: If you are over 40 and unused to regular exercise, switch exercises day by day. For instance, jog on Monday, Wednesday, and Friday; and cycle on Tuesday, Thursday, and Saturday.

Month_____   **Calculated Training Heart Rate**_____

Date	Exercise	Category	Time Spent (Minutes)	Ending Pulse Rate*

* If pulse is 10 beats too fast or slow, today's exercise cannot be used in the calculation for total time.

Month_____   **Total Monthly Time**

Totals: Category I   _____min. × 5/4 = _____
          Category II   _____min. × 1   = + _____
          Category III _____min. × 3/4 = + _____
          Total Adjusted Time = _____

You will probably maintain your present fitness level if you exercise at least 180 adjusted minutes a month. Fitness will improve slowly by exercising 360 adjusted minutes a month. Obviously, if you spend more time exercising you'll improve faster. Before you start another month . . .

1. Check your resting pulse.
2. If your resting pulse has decreased, you need to recalculate your training heart rate.
3. Check your measurements: Waist_____ Hips_____
                        Right Thigh_____ Right Upper Arm___
4. Weight_____

(People who are close to their correct weight will often notice an *increase* in weight when they exercise regularly. Do not be alarmed by this. You are adding muscle to your body as you exercise away the fat. If your measurements get slimmer, but your weight goes up, be assured that you are adding healthy muscle tissue to your body.)

Month_____ **Calculated Training Heart Rate**_____

Date	Exercise	Category	Time Spent (Minutes)	Ending Pulse Rate*

* If pulse is 10 beats too fast or slow, today's exercise cannot be used in the calculation for total time.

Month_____ **Total Monthly Time**

Totals: Category I   _____min. × 5/4 = _____
         Category II   _____min. × 1   = + _____
         Category III _____min. × 3/4 = + _____
                       Total Adjusted Time = _____

You will probably maintain your present fitness level if you exercise at least 180 adjusted minutes a month. Fitness will improve slowly by exercising 360 adjusted minutes a month. Obviously, if you spend more time exercising you'll improve faster. Before you start another month . . .

1. Check your resting pulse.
2. If your resting pulse has decreased, you need to recalculate your training heart rate.
3. Check your measurements: Waist_____ Hips_____
                            Right Thigh_____ Right Upper Arm____

4. Weight_____

(People who are close to their correct weight will often notice an *increase* in weight when they exercise regularly. Do not be alarmed by this. You are adding muscle to your body as you exercise away the fat. If your measurements get slimmer, but your weight goes up, be assured that you are adding healthy muscle tissue to your body.)

Month_____   **Calculated Training Heart Rate**_____

Date	Exercise	Category	Time Spent (Minutes)	Ending Pulse Rate*

* If pulse is 10 beats too fast or slow, today's exercise cannot be used in the calculation for total time.

Month_____   **Total Monthly Time**

Totals: Category I _____min. $\times$ 5/4 $=$ _____
         Category II _____min. $\times$ 1 $= +$ _____
         Category III _____min. $\times$ 3/4 $= +$ _____
                          Total Adjusted Time $=$ _____

You will probably maintain your present fitness level if you exercise at least 180 adjusted minutes a month. Fitness will improve slowly by exercising 360 adjusted minutes a month. Obviously, if you spend more time exercising you'll improve faster. Before you start another month . . .

1. Check your resting pulse.
2. If your resting pulse has decreased, you need to recalculate your training heart rate.
3. Check your measurements: Waist_____ Hips_____
                             Right Thigh_____ Right Upper Arm___
4. Weight_____

(People who are close to their correct weight will often notice an *increase* in weight when they exercise regularly. Do not be alarmed by this. You are adding muscle to your body as you exercise away the fat. If your measurements get slimmer, but your weight goes up, be assured that you are adding healthy muscle tissue to your body.)

Month_____   **Calculated Training Heart Rate**_____

Date	Exercise	Category	Time Spent (Minutes)	Ending Pulse Rate*

* If pulse is 10 beats too fast or slow, today's exercise cannot be used in the calculation for total time.

Month_____   **Total Monthly Time**

Totals: Category I   _____min. $\times$ 5/4 $=$ _____
           Category II   _____min. $\times$ 1 $=+$ _____
           Category III   _____min. $\times$ 3/4 $=+$ _____
                        Total Adjusted Time $=$ _____

You will probably maintain your present fitness level if you exercise at least 180 adjusted minutes a month. Fitness will improve slowly by exercising 360 adjusted minutes a month. Obviously, if you spend more time exercising you'll improve faster. Before you start another month . . .

1. Check your resting pulse.
2. If your resting pulse has decreased, you need to recalculate your training heart rate.
3. Check your measurements: Waist_____   Hips_____
                               Right Thigh_____   Right Upper Arm___
4. Weight_____

(People who are close to their correct weight will often notice an *increase* in weight when they exercise regularly. Do not be alarmed by this. You are adding muscle to your body as you exercise away the fat. If your measurements get slimmer, but your weight goes up, be assured that you are adding healthy muscle tissue to your body.)

Month_____   **Calculated Training Heart Rate**_____

Date	Exercise	Category	Time Spent (Minutes)	Ending Pulse Rate*

* If pulse is 10 beats too fast or slow, today's exercise cannot be used in the calculation for total time.

Month_____   **Total Monthly Time**

Totals: Category I   _____min. $\times$ 5/4 = _____
         Category II   _____min. $\times$ 1 = + _____
         Category III   _____min. $\times$ 3/4 = + _____
                        Total Adjusted Time = _____

You will probably maintain your present fitness level if you exercise at least 180 adjusted minutes a month. Fitness will improve slowly by exercising 360 adjusted minutes a month. Obviously, if you spend more time exercising you'll improve faster. Before you start another month . . .

1. Check your resting pulse.

2. If your resting pulse has decreased, you need to recalculate your training heart rate.

3. Check your measurements: Waist_____ Hips_____
                                Right Thigh_____ Right Upper Arm___

4. Weight_____

(People who are close to their correct weight will often notice an *increase* in weight when they exercise regularly. Do not be alarmed by this. You are adding muscle to your body as you exercise away the fat. If your measurements get slimmer, but your weight goes up, be assured that you are adding healthy muscle tissue to your body.)

Month_____   **Calculated Training Heart Rate**_____

Date	Exercise	Category	Time Spent (Minutes)	Ending Pulse Rate*

* If pulse is 10 beats too fast or slow, today's exercise cannot be used in the calculation for total time.

Month_____   **Total Monthly Time**

Totals: Category I   _____min. $\times$ 5/4 = _____
           Category II   _____min. $\times$ 1   = + _____
           Category III   _____min. $\times$ 3/4 = + _____

Total Adjusted Time = _____

You will probably maintain your present fitness level if you exercise at least 180 adjusted minutes a month. Fitness will improve slowly by exercising 360 adjusted minutes a month. Obviously, if you spend more time exercising you'll improve faster. Before you start another month . . .

1. Check your resting pulse.

2. If your resting pulse has decreased, you need to recalculate your training heart rate.

3. Check your measurements: Waist_____   Hips_____
                                 Right Thigh_____   Right Upper Arm___

4. Weight_____

(People who are close to their correct weight will often notice an *increase* in weight when they exercise regularly. Do not be alarmed by this. You are adding muscle to your body as you exercise away the fat. If your measurements get slimmer, but your weight goes up, be assured that you are adding healthy muscle tissue to your body.)

Month_____   **Calculated Training Heart Rate**_____

Date	Exercise	Category	Time Spent (Minutes)	Ending Pulse Rate*

* If pulse is 10 beats too fast or slow, today's exercise cannot be used in the calculation for total time.

Month_____   **Total Monthly Time**

Totals: Category I   _____min. $\times$ 5/4 = _____
             Category II   _____min. $\times$ 1   = + _____
             Category III   _____min. $\times$ 3/4 = + _____
                               Total Adjusted Time = _____

You will probably maintain your present fitness level if you exercise at least 180 adjusted minutes a month. Fitness will improve slowly by exercising 360 adjusted minutes a month. Obviously, if you spend more time exercising you'll improve faster. Before you start another month . . .

1. Check your resting pulse.
2. If your resting pulse has decreased, you need to recalculate your training heart rate.
3. Check your measurements: Waist_____   Hips_____
                                                  Right Thigh_____   Right Upper Arm___
4. Weight_____

(People who are close to their correct weight will often notice an *increase* in weight when they exercise regularly. Do not be alarmed by this. You are adding muscle to your body as you exercise away the fat. If your measurements get slimmer, but your weight goes up, be assured that you are adding healthy muscle tissue to your body.)

Month_____   **Calculated Training Heart Rate**_____

Date	Exercise	Category	Time Spent (Minutes)	Ending Pulse Rate*

* If pulse is 10 beats too fast or slow, today's exercise cannot be used in the calculation for total time.

Month_____   **Total Monthly Time**

Totals: Category I   _____min. $\times$ 5/4 = _____
         Category II   _____min. $\times$ 1   = +_____
         Category III   _____min. $\times$ 3/4 = +_____

Total Adjusted Time = _____

You will probably maintain your present fitness level if you exercise at least 180 adjusted minutes a month. Fitness will improve slowly by exercising 360 adjusted minutes a month. Obviously, if you spend more time exercising you'll improve faster. Before you start another month . . .

1. Check your resting pulse.

2. If your resting pulse has decreased, you need to recalculate your training heart rate.

3. Check your measurements: Waist_____   Hips_____
                             Right Thigh_____   Right Upper Arm___

4. Weight_____

(People who are close to their correct weight will often notice an *increase* in weight when they exercise regularly. Do not be alarmed by this. You are adding muscle to your body as you exercise away the fat. If your measurements get slimmer, but your weight goes up, be assured that you are adding healthy muscle tissue to your body.)

Month_____ **Calculated Training Heart Rate**_____

Date	Exercise	Category	Time Spent (Minutes)	Ending Pulse Rate*

* If pulse is 10 beats too fast or slow, today's exercise cannot be used in the calculation for total time.

Month_____ **Total Monthly Time**

Totals: Category I _____min. $\times$ 5/4 = _____
Category II _____min. $\times$ 1 = + _____
Category III _____min. $\times$ 3/4 = + _____
Total Adjusted Time = _____

You will probably maintain your present fitness level if you exercise at least 180 adjusted minutes a month. Fitness will improve slowly by exercising 360 adjusted minutes a month. Obviously, if you spend more time exercising you'll improve faster. Before you start another month . . .

1. Check your resting pulse.

2. If your resting pulse has decreased, you need to recalculate your training heart rate.

3. Check your measurements: Waist_____ Hips_____
Right Thigh_____ Right Upper Arm___

4. Weight_____

(People who are close to their correct weight will often notice an *increase* in weight when they exercise regularly. Do not be alarmed by this. You are adding muscle to your body as you exercise away the fat. If your measurements get slimmer, but your weight goes up, be assured that you are adding healthy muscle tissue to your body.)

Month_____   **Calculated Training Heart Rate**_____

Date	Exercise	Category	Time Spent (Minutes)	Ending Pulse Rate*

* If pulse is 10 beats too fast or slow, today's exercise cannot be used in the calculation for total time.

Month_____   **Total Monthly Time**

Totals: Category I   _____min. $\times$ 5/4 = _____
         Category II   _____min. $\times$ 1 = + _____
         Category III   _____min. $\times$ 3/4 = + _____
         Total Adjusted Time = _____

You will probably maintain your present fitness level if you exercise at least 180 adjusted minutes a month. Fitness will improve slowly by exercising 360 adjusted minutes a month. Obviously, if you spend more time exercising you'll improve faster. Before you start another month . . .

1. Check your resting pulse.

2. If your resting pulse has decreased, you need to recalculate your training heart rate.

3. Check your measurements: Waist_____ Hips_____
                            Right Thigh_____ Right Upper Arm___

4. Weight_____

(People who are close to their correct weight will often notice an *increase* in weight when they exercise regularly. Do not be alarmed by this. You are adding muscle to your body as you exercise away the fat. If your measurements get slimmer, but your weight goes up, be assured that you are adding healthy muscle tissue to your body.)

Month_____   **Calculated Training Heart Rate**_____

Date	Exercise	Category	Time Spent (Minutes)	Ending Pulse Rate*

* If pulse is 10 beats too fast or slow, today's exercise cannot be used in the calculation for total time.

Month_____   **Total Monthly Time**

Totals: Category I   _____min. $\times$ 5/4 = _____
           Category II   _____min. $\times$ 1   = + _____
           Category III   _____min. $\times$ 3/4 = + _____
                        Total Adjusted Time = _____

You will probably maintain your present fitness level if you exercise at least 180 adjusted minutes a month. Fitness will improve slowly by exercising 360 adjusted minutes a month. Obviously, if you spend more time exercising you'll improve faster. Before you start another month . . .

1. Check your resting pulse.
2. If your resting pulse has decreased, you need to recalculate your training heart rate.
3. Check your measurements: Waist_____   Hips_____
                                Right Thigh_____   Right Upper Arm___
4. Weight_____

(People who are close to their correct weight will often notice an *increase* in weight when they exercise regularly. Do not be alarmed by this. You are adding muscle to your body as you exercise away the fat. If your measurements get slimmer, but your weight goes up, be assured that you are adding healthy muscle tissue to your body.)

Month_____ **Calculated Training Heart Rate**_____

Date	Exercise	Category	Time Spent (Minutes)	Ending Pulse Rate*

* If pulse is 10 beats too fast or slow, today's exercise cannot be used in the calculation for total time.

Month_____ **Total Monthly Time**

Totals: Category I _____ min. $\times$ 5/4 = _____
Category II _____ min. $\times$ 1 = + _____
Category III _____ min. $\times$ 3/4 = + _____
Total Adjusted Time = _____

You will probably maintain your present fitness level if you exercise at least 180 adjusted minutes a month. Fitness will improve slowly by exercising 360 adjusted minutes a month. Obviously, if you spend more time exercising you'll improve faster. Before you start another month . . .

1. Check your resting pulse.
2. If your resting pulse has decreased, you need to recalculate your training heart rate.
3. Check your measurements: Waist_____ Hips_____
   Right Thigh_____ Right Upper Arm___
4. Weight_____

(People who are close to their correct weight will often notice an *increase* in weight when they exercise regularly. Do not be alarmed by this. You are adding muscle to your body as you exercise away the fat. If your measurements get slimmer, but your weight goes up, be assured that you are adding healthy muscle tissue to your body.)